C000096315

KETO INTERMITTENT FASTING

THE SIMPLE AND POWERFUL
STEP-BY-STEP METHOD TO
UNLOCK THE SECRETS OF A
LASTING HEALTHY LIFESTYLE!
(WITH RECIPES AND MEAL
PLAN)

JASON RAMOS

TABLE OF CONTENTS

TABLE OF CONTENTS

TABLE OF CONTENTS

TABLE OF CONTENTS

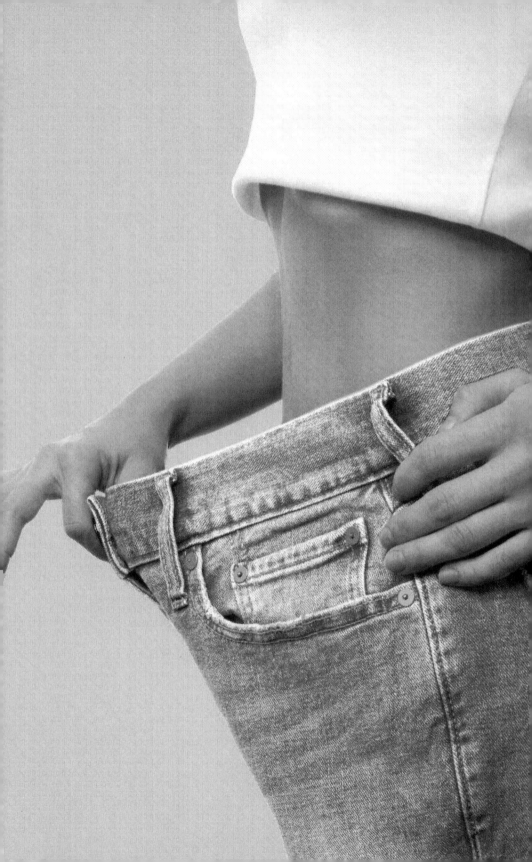

INTRODUCTION

First off, I would like to thank you for choosing this book. I hope that you find it helpful and that it will help you reach your goals of weight loss and reversing your diabetes.

First off, we will go over the reversibility and prevention of diabetes, and the best way to use this book. This will help to give you a good understanding of what you can expect this book to cover.

Then we will go deeper into the subject of diseases and healthy lifestyles. This chapter will help you look at your life to see how healthy or unhealthy it is so that you can figure out where you need to make changes.

Next, we will start to look at how the body works. This will look further into diabetes and how type 1 and type 2 are different. We will also cover the subject of insulin and what it does for your body. We will also discuss energy for your cells and how your body stores fat.

Then we will get into the information about fasting. I know that's what you really came here for, and I promise it will be worth the wait. Here we will go over the basics of fasting and what it means.

Next, we will look at the different schedules that you can choose from. Intermittent fasting isn't one-size-fits-all, so you can figure out which schedule works best for you.

Then we will look at how the ketogenic diet and intermittent fasting work together. This has become a very popular diet, and people tend to start fasting naturally on this diet. This doesn't mean that you have to follow a keto diet to fast, but that is an option.

You will find information about food and drinks. This will go over what nutrients and foods you should aim to eat when you are fasting. This is also where you will find 60 recipes that you can use.

Next, we will talk about how fasting can be different for women. Some people advise women not to fast at all because it affects their body differently than it does men, but women can still safely fast.

We will also go talk about exercising while fasting. Again, some people don't think this is safe, but it is as long as you are smart about it.

Lastly, we will go over some frequently asked questions so that you can start fasting with confidence.

FOREWORD

Using this book is very straight forward. First, I would suggest just reading through the whole book. Don't worry about fully and completely understanding the topics at hand, just read through it and try to learn as much as you can. Then, go back and reread anything you are confused about. The main thing you want to make sure you understand is the different types of fasting, and how to make sure you don't do yourself more harm than good.

Once you feel you are ready, pick one of the schedules that mesh well with your time and give it a try. Remember, the first few days may be difficult. Your body is used to getting food all day long, so not feeding it as often is going to upset it, but persevere. You will get used to it.

Type 2 diabetes is a long-term condition that can be very serious. It usually happens to adults, but recently, it has become more common in children since obesity rates continue to rise in people of all ages. There are several factors that contribute to this horrible disease. The biggest risk factor is being obese or overweight.

Type 2 diabetes could be life-threatening. If it is treated very carefully, it is possible to manage it and possibly reverse it.

Before a doctor diagnoses you with diabetes, there will be a time where blood sugar levels will be high but they won't be high enough to get diagnosed with diabetes. This is called prediabetes. About 70 percent of all the people who have been diagnosed with prediabetes will eventually develop type 2 diabetes. This isn't saying that you will get diabetes. You can change your lifestyle to where you won't go into diabetes.

There are factors that you won't be able to change like your past behaviors, age, or genes, but there are actions you can do to reduce your risk of getting diabetes.

This disease impacts the way your body metabolizes sugar. Your pancreas will either produce enough insulin or your body becomes resistant to it. This will cause glucose to begin building up in the blood. This is known as hyperglycemia.

There are many symptoms of type 2 diabetes if it goes untreated. These could be:

- Dark blotches on the skin

- Blurred vision

- Skin infections that heal very slowly

- Losing weight even though you are eating more

- Hungry a lot

- Fatigue

- Excessive urination and thirst

To treat type 2 diabetes, you have to use insulin or medications if needed and monitor your blood sugar levels. Your doctor will also want you to lose weight by following a specific diet plan and exercising. Some medications for diabetes might help you lose some weight which, in turn, could help reverse your diabetes.

If you begin to eat healthier, lose weight, and exercise more, you could reduce some symptoms. Weight loss is the main factor in people who have been able to reverse their diabetes because having excess fat in the body will affect how much insulin is produced and used.

In one study done in 2011, 11 people who had type 2 diabetes reduced their intake of calories for eight weeks and this helped reverse their condition. Researchers found that this was only one small sample and the volunteers had only had diabetes for a few years.

Other studies have shown that bariatric surgery could reverse type 2 diabetes, too. This is one of only a few ways to actually reverse diabetes for a long time.

There are other ways you can lose weight to help reduce your symptoms. Committing to changing your diet and getting regular exercise might be all you need to do.

Start Moving

Beginning an exercise routine is essential for your health. It could also help you lose some weight and your symptoms will begin to reverse. Speak with your physician before you make any plans and remember the following:

- Keep a snack with you so you will be covered if your blood sugar drops when you are working out.

- Keep a check on your blood sugar at all times. Check it before, during, and after you have exercised.

- When you walk, make it a brisk walk. Walking fast is a great way to exercise. Brisk walking is easy and doesn't take any equipment.

- Begin slowly. If you haven't exercised in a long time, begin small with some short walks. Slowly increase the intensity and duration.

Watch What You Eat

You need to improve what you eat. This can help you lose some weight which will, in turn, help you manage your symptoms and could possibly reverse your diabetes. Your physician could help you plan a balanced and healthy diet or they might send you to see a dietitian.

This diet can help you manage or even reverse your diabetes and should include:

- Limited sweets

- Limited alcohol

- Lean proteins like beans, soy, low-fat dairy, fish, and poultry

- Whole grains

- Various fresh vegetables and fruits

- Healthy fats

- Reduced calories

Some doctors are beginning to support the ketogenic diet to help stabilize blood sugar and lose weight. For you to figure out what your carbohydrate intake needs to be, work with your dietitian or doctor. Think about your dietary preferences and metabolic goals when figuring out which diet you should do.

It is possible to reverse your type 2 diabetes but it takes commitment, regular exercise, healthy eating, and meal planning. If you are able to do these things and lose some weight, you might be able to reverse your diabetes and everything it causes.

Difference Between Type 2 and Type 1 Diabetes

Type 1 and type 2 diabetes are similar but type 1 normally develops during childhood and isn't related to diet or weight. The causes behind type 1 diabetes aren't known but the most risk factors seem to be family history and genetics.

If you have been diagnosed with type 1 diabetes, your pancreas doesn't make enough insulin. You have to inject insulin in order to metabolize your glucose. It can be managed, but there isn't a cure and there isn't any way to reverse it. The symptoms of type 1 are exactly the same as the ones for type 2 diabetes.

Both could cause serious complication if it isn't treated or managed and these could include:

- Hearing problems
- Osteoporosis
- Foot infections that could lead to an amputation
- Mouth and skin infections
- Kidney damage
- Blindness and vision problems
- Atherosclerosis
- Nerve damage
- Heart disease

Here are some ways to help you stay away from being diagnosed with diabetes:

- Drink tea or coffee

Water needs to be your go-to beverage, but research shows that adding tea or coffee to your diet could help you avoid diabetes. These studies show that drinking coffee daily can reduce your risk of type 2 diabetes by between 8 and 54 percent. The largest effect was seen in people who drank more coffee each day.

Another study shows that coffee and tea found the same results and the largest reduction was in women and men who are overweight. Tea and coffee have antioxidants that are called polyphenols that could help protect you against diabetes. Green tea has unique antioxidant compounds that are called epigallocatechin gallate or EGCG that can reduce the release of blood sugar and increase insulin sensitivity.

- Lower how much processed foods you eat

A good step that you could take to improve your health is to lower your consumption of processed foods. These have been linked to all kinds of health problems like diabetes, obesity, and heart disease. Studies show that eating less prepackaged foods that contain a lot of additives, vegetable oils, and refined grains could help lower a person's diabetes risk.

This is because of the protective effects of foods such as veggies, fruits, nuts, and other plant-based foods. One study has found that diets that are high in processed foods can up a person's risk of getting diabetes by 30 percent. When you include nutritious foods, it can help reduce this risk.

- Increase your Vitamin D intake

Vitamin D can help control your blood sugar. Studies show that people who don't get enough vitamin D have a larger risk of diabetes. Many health organizations say you should keep a vitamin D blood level around 30 ng/ml.

One study found that people who had high blood levels of vitamin D were 43 percent less likely to get type 2 diabetes than ones with lower blood levels.

Another study looked at children from Finland who took supplements that contained vitamin D. The children who had the vitamin D supplements had about a 78 percent lower risk of developing type 1 diabetes than the children who didn't take any supplements.

Controlled studies show that if people who are vitamin D deficient take supplements, their blood sugar levels will regulate, their insulin-producing cells will improve, and it reduces their risk of diabetes.

You can find vitamin D in certain food sources like cod liver oil and fatty fish. Being out in the sun will also increase the level of vitamin D in the blood. For most people, taking a supplement of 2,000 to 4,000 IUs daily will help achieve and maintain the right level of vitamin D.

- High Fiber Diets

Eating a lot of fiber is beneficial for weight management and gut health. Studies performed on prediabetic patients who are elderly and obese showed it can help keep blood sugar and insulin levels low.

Fiber is able to be divided into two categories: soluble and insoluble. Insoluble fiber won't absorb water where soluble fiber does. When water and soluble fiber reach the digestive tract, it forms a gel that will slow down how fast food gets absorbed. This can cause blood sugar levels to rise slower.

Insoluble fiber can reduce blood sugar levels along with decreasing the risk of diabetes. The way it works isn't clear.

Most plant-based foods will contain fiber even though some will have more than others.

- Stay away from being sedentary

It is important to stop being sedentary if you want to stay away from diabetes. If you don't get very much physical activity and you sit for most of your day, you are leading a sedentary life.

Studies have shown consistency between the risk of diabetes and sedentary behaviors. People who spent the majority of their day living a sedentary lifestyle have an increased risk of 91 percent of developing diabetes.

Changing your sedentary behavior is as easy as standing up at your desk and walking around for a few minutes each hour. It is very hard to reverse habits that are extremely hardwired.

You have to set achievable and realistic goals like standing while you are on the phone or walking up the stairs rather than taking the elevator. If you can commit to these concrete but easy actions, it might be the best way to reverse your sedentary habits.

- Portion control

It doesn't matter what diet you decide to follow, what is important is to stay away from large portions of food to lower your risk of diabetes. This very is important if you are already overweight. Eating large portions of food at one time can cause higher insulin and blood sugar levels in people who are at risk of diabetes.

Decreasing your portion sizes might help prevent this kind of response. One study done in men who are prediabetic found the ones who reduced their portion sizes and practiced other healthy behaviors had almost a 50 percent lower risk of developing diabetes.

Other studies looked at various weight loss methods in prediabetic people but the ones who practiced portion control actually lowered their insulin and blood sugar levels significantly in 12 weeks.

• Stop smoking

It has been proven that smoking can cause or contribute to several serious health conditions like cancer of the digestive tract, prostate, breast, and lung, emphysema, and heart disease. Research also shows a link between exposure to second-hand smoke and smoking to type 2 diabetes. In several studies, smoking increased the risk of diabetes by 44 percent in an average smoker and 61 percent in others who smoked over 20 cigarettes each day.

One study looked at middle-aged men who were smokers but had quit. After just five years, their risk had already reduced by 13 percent, and in 20 years, they had the same risks as people who hadn't ever smoked.

Research states that even if the men gained some weight after they quit, after being smoke-free for many years, their risk was a lot lower than if they had continued to smoke.

- If you are obese or overweight, lose some weight

Even though everybody who develops type 2 diabetes isn't obese or overweight, most of them are. People who are prediabetic usually carry their excess weight around their midsection. This fat is around the abdominal organs such as the liver. This is known as visceral fat. This fat will promote inflammation and insulin resistance which ups your risk of diabetes. Even if you can lose a small amount of weight, it could help reduce this risk. Studies have shown that the more you can lose, the more benefits you will gain. One study showed that for each kilogram of weight prediabetics lost, their risk of being diagnosed with diabetes dropped by 16 percent. Some even had a maximum reduction of 96 percent.

There are several healthy options to help you lose weight like vegetarian, paleo, Mediterranean, and low-carb diets. Picking a way of eating that you can stick with for a long time is the most important part of helping you keep the weight off.

One study found that overweight people whose insulin and blood sugar levels did decrease after they lost weight experienced an elevation of these after they gained back some of the weight they had lost.

- Make water your main beverage

Water is the most natural beverage that you can drink. Drinking water most of the time will help you stay away from drinks that are high in preservatives, sugars, and questionable ingredients. Beverages that are full of sugar like punch and soda have shown to increase the risk of both latent autoimmune diabetes of adults (LADA) and type 2 diabetes.

LADA is a variation of type 1 diabetes that happens in people who are over 18 years old. It doesn't have acute symptoms like type 1 diabetes in children. It develops slowly and requires more treatments as the disease gets worse.

One large study looked at 2,800 people and their risk of developing diabetes. People who drank more than two servings of sugary beverages each day had a 99 percent increased risk of being diagnosed with LADA and a 20 percent risk of getting type 2 diabetes. Researchers also noted that fruit juice or artificially sweetened beverages weren't good to help prevent diabetes.

Drinking a lot of water might give these results. Studies have shown that drinking more water might lead to better insulin response and better blood sugar control. One study showed that adults who are overweight that replaced their sodas with water while following a diet program experienced a reduction in insulin levels and fasting blood sugar and a decrease in insulin resistance.

• Exercise Regularly

Exercising regularly might help prevent diabetes. When you exercise, it can increase the insulin sensitivity of the cells. When you exercise, you don't need as much insulin to keep your blood sugar levels in control. One study about prediabetic people found that moderate-intensity exercise could increase insulin sensitivity by about 51 percent, whereas high-intensity exercise increases it by 85 percent. This effect only happened on days they exercised.

Most types of physical activity can reduce blood sugar and insulin resistance in people who are obese, overweight, and prediabetic. These could include strength training, high-intensity interval training, and aerobic exercises.

Exercising more frequently can lead to improvements in insulin function and response. One study found that burning over 2,000 calories each week through exercises was needed to reach these results. It is best to pick a physical activity that you like doing, can do regularly, and you know you will stick with for a long time.

Eating the correct foods and changing your lifestyle behaviors that will promote healthy insulin and blood sugar levels will give you a great chance at staying away from diabetes.

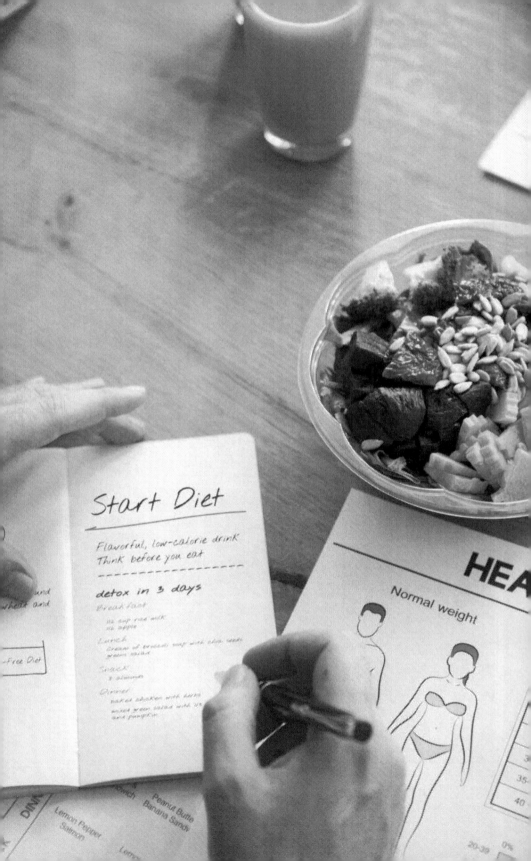

BEFORE YOU START

The average American can expect to live to around the age of 77. Surely, this isn't the best we can do? Are there ways we can expand our lifespan? Records show that the oldest person in the United States was 122 years old when they passed away.

In order to be able to answer questions like these, you have to have some understanding of what happens to the body as it ages. As humans, have we been trained to live for a certain number of years or does our body wear out? There are theories people have as to the reason we live as long as we do.

First, it is believed that our genes determine the amount of time we live. It says that genes or several genes let our bodies know how long we are allowed to live. If you had the ability to change those genes, you would be able to live as long as you wanted to.

The second gene says that with time, your DNA and body will get so damaged that it can't function properly anymore. It is basically saying that the length of our lives is simply caused by the changes within our DNA. All of these changes continue to add up until there is too much damage for your body to bear, and then you die.

And it really does matter as to which theory is correct because it will determine how we are able to push the limits in aging. If our genes actually hold the number to the age we live, then in order to increase how long we live, we might be able to change those genes. But if our age is based on all the damage we have done to our bodies during our lifetime, we can try to lessen the damage and try to live longer.

So, which of these theories are right? Reality is a combination of both of these ideas. During the past ten years, scientists have found some evidence that supports both theories.

Research that was done in worms showed that mutating specific genes could increase our life about four-fold. This would come out to about 300 years for humans. The findings coincide with the idea that people have genes that determine the length of time we live.

If the body uses those genes to fix damage due to aging, then that means the second model is correct. In one disease known as Werner's syndrome, genes mutated to cause people to age faster. The mutated gene is believed to be a part of the process of maintaining DNA.

There were other studies that found that not eating as much could increase an animal's life. Even though the reason for increasing the length of our life isn't clear right now, scientists have proposed that it involves decreasing cellular and DNA damage. Other studies suggest that cells can only divide so many times. This is due to the DNA that lives at the end of the chromosomes, which are called telomeres, getting shorter every time it divides. When all of this runs out, the cell dies.

You've probably figured out that the understanding process is challenging. There are a number of scientists that are consumed by the subject, so research is continuing to make quick progress.

It doesn't matter whether you want to lower your odds of getting a disease, losing weight, or getting stronger, you need to take some time to find your baseline. You can't track your progress if you don't know where you are starting from.

Before you dive right in, look at these circumstances and measurements. They will help you understand your current health status so you can move forward knowing what you need to know.

- Waist and Weight

The number on your scale isn't the only thing that matters when you want to be healthier. It can give you some important clues about your risk for certain conditions like arthritis, cancer, heart disease, and a lot more.

In order to know if your weight is healthy for you, get on your scale. Once you have that number, use a calculator to find your BMI. This uses your weight and height. 150 pounds will mean something extremely different to somebody who is five feet tall as compared to someone who is six feet tall. Having a BMI between 18.5 to 24.9 is in the normal range.

Now, find a tape measure. Even if you have a normal BMI, if you have extra fat on your midsection, it means you risk more of getting heart disease and type 2 diabetes. A healthy waist measurement for a woman is about 35 inches where a normal measurement for a man would be about 40 inches.

- Exercise

Doing any type of activity is better than doing nothing. Most adults need to try to get around 2.5 hours of moderate-intensity activity every week. If you do exercises in small spurts instead of longer workouts at the gym, that is perfectly fine. Think about wearing a pedometer for a week so you will be able to see your normal activity level. Most experts say you need to get about 10,000 steps daily and this equals to around five miles.

- Partners

You need to have a doctor that you feel comfortable with for your checkups and to contact when you have certain concerns about your health. If you do, great. If not, find one. This is your main priority right now. Your doctor needs to keep you updated on tests such as colonoscopies, mammograms, and checking your cholesterol.

You might need to see a specialist from time to time like an allergist, cardiologist, or endocrinologist for any health issues that might come up. Social support is also important. You will stay motivated and on track if you have family and friends who share and encourage your goals.

- Mood

Mental health is as important as physical health. These two go together like carrots and hummus. Poor mental health could zap your focus or energy and could raise the chance of heart disease. If you can't figure out how to stop feeling overwhelmed, down, or stressed, it might be time to find a mental health professional to help you.

- Sleep

The average adult needs about seven to nine hours of sleep nightly. Everybody is different so you have to listen to your body. If you get sleepy when driving, going about your day, or if you have to drink coffee to get through the day, you probably aren't getting enough sleep. The first thing to do is to begin tracking your sleep. Apps and devices might give you more data than journaling or writing it down.

- Diet

All those tiny little bites that you steal from your children's plate or that extra doughnut at the morning meeting are easy to look over, but with time, they will add up.

To be sure you are paying attention to what you are putting into your mouth, spend a couple of days writing down every single thing you eat. You could use an app on your phone or write it down on paper. You need to be very specific. Instead of writing down "potato chips", you should put "25 baked potato chips with ¼ cup ranch dip." You could add notes about how you were feeling, who you were with, where you were, or what you were doing to help you see any patterns that might be developing.

When you are making notes about what you eat, don't forget to also add in what you are drinking. Energy drinks and sugary soft drinks are a huge source of calories that could cause you to become obese.

Don't go thirsty. An average adult will need no less than eight cups of water daily to remain hydrated. If you see you are having problems drinking enough, track your water in your food diary.

What about alcohol? If you are a woman, you shouldn't consume more than one drink daily and men, no more than two.

- Blood Numbers

If you don't know your blood sugar, blood pressure, and cholesterol, you need to go see your doctor. For healthy adults, the numbers should be:

o Fasting blood glucose: under 100 mg/dL

o Total cholesterol: under 200 mg/dL

o Blood pressure: under 120/80

Your doctor might have target numbers that are different depending on any conditions or your medical situation.

Diabetes

What happens if you have already been diagnosed with diabetes? Let's look at what diabetes is first. Diabetes mellitus refers to diseases that change the way your body uses glucose. Glucose plays a very important part in your body since it is one of the main sources of energy the cells use that form your tissues and muscles. The brain can only use glucose, and one other thing, as energy.

The main cause of diabetes is different for each type. It doesn't matter which type you have, it can create too much sugar within the blood. With the increase of sugar in the blood, many serious health problems can be created.

Type 1 and type 2 are chronic diabetes. Gestational and prediabetes are both reversible. Prediabetes occurs when the blood sugar levels are elevated but they haven't reached the level of diabetes, yet. Gestational diabetes happens when a woman is pregnant but usually resolves once the baby is born.

- Seeing Your Doctor

o Once you have been diagnosed with diabetes, you will need to continue to see your doctor until your blood sugar is stabilized.

o If you see any diabetic symptoms, get in touch with your doctor. The sooner you can get diagnosed, the sooner you will be able to start treatments.

Causes

In order to understand diabetes, you have to know how the body is supposed to process glucose.

- What Insulin Does

Insulin is a hormone that the pancreas secretes into the bloodstream. It circulates and allows the sugar to go into your cells. Insulin helps lower how much sugar goes into the bloodstream. When your blood sugar levels get lower, your pancreas won't secrete as much insulin.

- Type 1 Diabetes Causes

What causes type 1 diabetes isn't clearly known. What we do know is that the immune system starts destroying and attacking pancreatic cells, which produce insulin. This will leave you with either no or little insulin. Rather than cells getting to use it, the sugar starts to build up in the blood.

It is believed that type 1 could be due to a combination of environmental factors and genetic susceptibility although what exactly the factors aren't clear. Weight isn't thought to be a cause of type 1 diabetes.

- Type 2 and Prediabetes Causes

When it comes to type 2 and prediabetes, the cells become resistant to insulin, which causes the pancreas not to be able to create enough insulin to work through the resistance. Rather than being used by the cells, where it becomes energy, the sugar stays in the blood.

It isn't clear what exactly happens, even though it is thought that environmental factors and genetics play roles here, too. Being obese or overweight is one of the causes of type 2 diabetes, but that doesn't mean you have to be overweight to develop type 2 diabetes.

- Gestational Diabetes

While a woman is pregnant, the placenta will produce hormones so that the pregnancy can be sustained. These hormones will sometimes cause your cells to become resistant to insulin.

Normally, the pancreas is able to respond by creating more insulin that is needed to work through this resistance. There may be times that the pancreas won't be able to keep up. If this happens, there won't be enough glucose in the cells because it will all be in the blood. This, in turn, causes gestational diabetes.

Complications

The long-term complications of diabetes usually develop slowly. The less your blood sugar is controlled and the longer you have diabetes, the higher your risk is of developing complications. Eventually, these complications might become life-threatening or disabling. Some possible complications are:

1. Depression: People who have diabetes will sometimes end up developing depression. This can play a part in how well you manage your diabetes.

2. Alzheimer's disease: Type 2 diabetes has the ability to increase your risk of developing Alzheimer's disease. If you have poor blood sugar, the higher your risk will be. Even though researchers have come up with a few theories as to how these diseases are connected, none of them have actually been proven.

3. Hearing problems: People who have diabetes usually develop hearing problems.

4. Skin conditions: If you have diabetes, you might have skin problems like fungal or bacterial infections.

5. Foot problems: Poor blood circulation or nerve damage to the feet can increase the odds of developing problems in your feet. If they aren't treated, blisters or cuts could end up becoming badly infected, which usually will not heal correctly. This can end up leading to gangrene, which could mean that the leg, foot, or toe has to be amputated.

6. Retinopathy: Having diabetes has the ability to damage the retina's blood vessels, which is what causes diabetic retinopathy, which could end up leading to blindness. Diabetes also increases a person's risk of developing other types of serious vision problems like glaucoma and cataracts.

7. Nephropathy: The kidneys are home to millions of tiny little clusters of blood vessels known as glomeruli that work to filter out waste in the blood. Diabetes has the ability to damage this system. Severe damage will then cause irreversible kidney disease or it could cause

kidney failure. This could mean that the person has to undergo a kidney transplant or dialysis.

8. Neuropathy: Too much sugar could hurt the walls of the capillaries, which are small blood vessels that help to nourish the nerves, especially those that are in your legs. This will end up causing pain, numbness, burning, or tingling that will typically start at the tips of fingers or toes and will then start to spread up.

9. Cardiovascular disease: Diabetes can drastically increase the risk of many cardiovascular problems; this could include narrowing of the arteries (atherosclerosis), stroke, chest pain, heart attack, and coronary artery disease. When a person has diabetes, it puts them at a higher risk of having a stroke or heart disease.

- Gestational diabetes

The majority of women who develop gestational diabetes will end up having healing babies. But if the blood sugar levels are left uncontrolled or untreated could cause problems for your baby and you.

The baby might develop complications because of gestational diabetes, including:

o Death: If your gestational diabetes goes untreated, it could result in your baby dying shortly after or right before birth.

o Type 2 diabetes later: If the mom had gestational diabetes, it puts the baby at a higher risk of being diagnosed with type 2 diabetes later on in life.

o Low blood sugar: Some babies born to moms who had gestational diabetes will have low blood sugar as a newborn because they produced so much insulin. Feeding promptly of glucose solution given intravenously could return the blood sugar back to normal.

o Excess growth: The extra glucose could go into the placenta which can cause the baby's pancreas to create more insulin. This may mean that the baby ends up being very large. Most babies like this will require a C-section.

The mom might develop complications because of gestational diabetes, including:

o Gestational diabetes in another pregnancy: If you develop gestational diabetes with one pregnancy, then you are more likely to develop it with the next one as well. It also places you at a greater risk of developing type 2 diabetes.

o Preeclampsia: This is a condition that is characterized by swelling of the feet and legs, too much protein in the urine, and high blood pressure. Preeclampsia could cause some serious and life-threatening problems for the baby and mom.

Prevention

You can't prevent type 1 diabetes. All of the same healthy choices can help to take care of gestation, type 2, and prediabetes and it can help to prevent the development of them as well:

- Lose some weight: When a person is overweight, simply losing seven percent of their weight can help to lower their risk of developing any form of diabetes.

This should not be something that a woman should try when she is pregnant, though. Speak with your doctor about your weight concerns and find out what would be healthy for you during your pregnancy.

Your weight should be kept in a healthy range, so try to focus on permanent changes in exercising more and improving the way you eat. You can motivate yourself by keeping in mind all the benefits of losing weight like improved self-esteem, more energy, and a healthier heart.

- Exercise: Try to get 30 minutes of moderate activity daily. Go swimming, ride your bike, take a walk, whatever you like to do, just get out and do it. If you can't make time to work out for 30 minutes straight, do small sessions throughout the day.

- Eat healthier: Pick foods that are low in calories and fat and high in fiber. Try to focus on whole grains, vegetables, and fruits. Choose a variety so you won't get bored.

Medication might be an option for you. Diabetic drugs like metformin might lower your risk of type 2 diabetes. A healthy lifestyle is the best way to go when it comes to lowering your diabetes risk. To make sure that you aren't at risk of developing type 2 diabetes, or if you already have it, make sure that you check your blood sugar levels once a year.

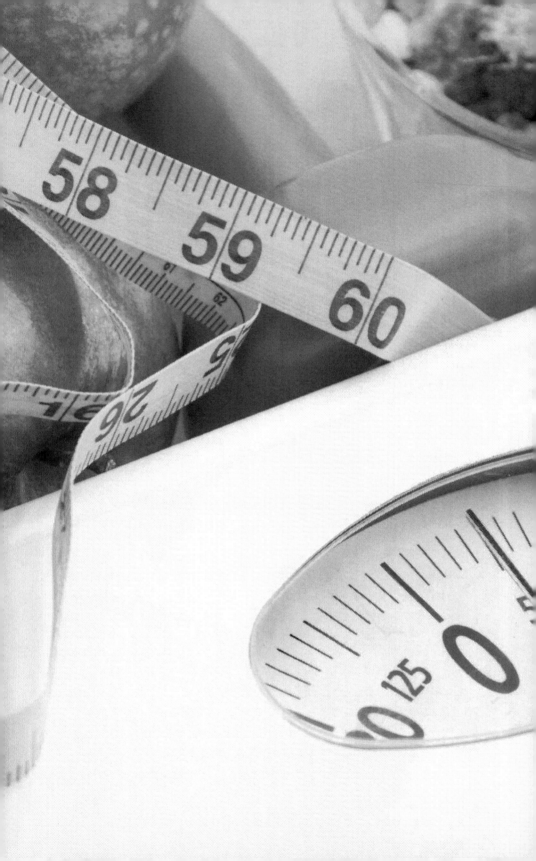

HOW MY BODY WORKS

Cells manage many functions within their tiny package. They grow, move, and housekeep. Many of these functions take energy. How do cells get their energy? How can they make use of this energy in an effective way?

Where Does Cell Energy Come From?

Just like humans, cells can't make their own energy. They have to locate a form of energy in their environment. Humans are able to find different substances such as fossil fuel to use as energy in their cares, cells, business, and homes. Pretty much every plant cell, photosynthetic prokaryotes, and algae will use the sun as their main source of energy so that they can make complex organic molecules that other types of the cells need to have for energy in order to aid with growth, reproduction, and metabolism.

There are many different forms of cell nutrients, like fats and sugars. In order for the cell to receive energy, the different molecules must move through the cell's membrane that works like a barrier, but not one that is impassable. Much like the outside walls of buildings and houses, the membrane of the plasma is considered to be semi-permeable.

It works much in the same way as to how the windows and doors in a wall allow necessary things into the house. The different proteins are able to move through the membrane of the cell which allows different molecules to move into the cell, even though they could need a little bit of energy to actually accomplish this.

How Do Cells Change Nutrients into Energy that Can be Used?

Complex food molecules are things like proteins, sugars, and fats, and they are the best sources of energy that you can provide your cells because most of the energy that forms all of these different molecules is stored in chemical bonds that bind all of them together. Scientists are able to measure the energy that is found in food by using what is known as a bomb calorimeter. When this technique is used, the food is placed in the calorimeter and it heats it up until it has been burned. The heat that is released through this is the same as the energy that food holds.

Cells don't actually work like this. They burn their energy in a single large reaction. The cells will then release all of the energy that is within the food molecules through some type of oxidation reaction. Oxidation is a type of chemical reaction where the electrons are taken out of one molecule and then moved into another one. All of the energy and composition content is changed in the acceptor and donor molecules. The molecules in food act like the electron donor. When the oxidation reactions happen to breakdown food, the products of all of these reactions will not have as much energy content than the original molecule. Electron acceptor molecules grab hold of the energy that was lost during the oxidative reaction and then is stored to later use. Eventually, all of the carbon atoms from the food molecules are completely oxidized once it reaches the end of the reactive chain. This is all then released as carbon dioxide waste.

Cells don't use what energy is created from the oxidation reactions once it is released. Rather, it gets transformed into small molecules that are full of energy like nicotinamide adenine dinucleotide or NADH and ATP that gets used in the cell to help metabolism and created new parts. This chemical energy is used by enzymes to accelerate or catalyze chemical reactions within the cell that normally go extremely slowly. Enzymes don't force reactions to go forward if it is unable to perform this action without a catalyst. They will, instead, reduce the energy that is needed for the reaction to start.

Pathways Used by Cells

A cell's chosen pathway is dependent upon whether or not it is a prokaryote or eukaryote. Cells that are eukaryotic will use three processes to change the energy within a chemical bond of molecules into something that is more usable, which tend to be energy-rich carrier molecules. ATP is the largest energy carrier within a cell. This molecule is constructed of a nitrogen base, three phosphate groups, and ribose sugar. Adenosine is the ribose sugar plus the adenine.

The mitochondrial membrane's transport chain isn't the only thing that is able to generate energy inside a cell. Within photosynthetic cells, chloroplasts hold the electron transport chain that makes use of the sun's energy. Even when prokaryotes don't have chloroplast or mitochondria, they have other types of electrons that yield energy in their membranes in order to create energy.

Energy Reserve in Cells

Eukaryotic cells, when plenty of energy exists, will force larger molecules to hold onto the extra energy. All of the fats and sugars will then be placed into reservoirs in the cells. There are some that are even big enough that they can be seen in electron micrographs.

Both animal and plant cells store energy by putting glucose into fat pathways. Every single storage mechanism is important because cells have to have quick and slow energy deposits. They store fats within droplets inside of the cytoplasm. Adipose cells are formed only for storage because they have bigger fat droplets. Humans will always have enough fat stored in order to provide their cells energy for many weeks.

Cells have to have the energy to do the tasks it needs to in order to survive. Starting with the energy sources they get from the environment like food molecules and sunlight. Eukaryotic cells make molecules like NADH and ATP through pathways including oxidative phosphorylation, citric acid cycle, glycolysis, and photosynthesis. Any extra energy gets stored in larger molecules like lipids and polysaccharides.

The Way Our Bodies Burn Fat

Most of us might be thinking about "burning some fat" so we can feel better in our bathing suits at the pool or the beach. What does this mean?

Fat cells exist just to store energy. The body expands the number of these cells and how big the fat cells are to accommodate the extra energy from foods that are high in calories. It will even begin to deposit fat in our liver, muscles, and other organs to make space to store all the extra energy from our calorie-laden diets.

Fat storage historically worked well for us. The energy was stored as fatty acids that got released into the bloodstream for fuel to be used by organs and muscles when they had to run from a predator or there wasn't food available. Fat storage was actually a survival mechanism for certain situations. People whose bodies stored fat could survive for longer time spans without food and had extra energy for environments that were hostile.

When did you ever have to run from a predator? Now, there is an overabundance of food and we all have very safe living conditions. Most people have a lot of fat stored. About 1/3 of the adults in the United States are obese.

The biggest problem with excess fat is that fat cells, called adipocytes, don't function normally. They release energy at a very slow rate and store it at an extremely high rate. These enlarged, extra fat cells produce huge amounts of various hormones. These hormones will increase inflammation, contribute to disease, and slow down metabolism. This complicated process of dysfunction and excess fat is known as adiposopathy. It makes treating obesity extremely difficult.

When you start and maintain a new exercise routine and begin limiting calories, the body will do two things in order to burn fat. First, it will use any energy that is stored in fat cells to fuel these new activities. Second, it will stop storing so much fat.

The brain will signal the fat cells to release the fatty acid molecules into the bloodstream. The heart, lungs, and muscles grab hold of these fatty acids, tear them apart, and use the energy stored to do their activities. What little bit remains get discarded through the breath as the outgoing carbon dioxide or through the urine. This will leave the fat cell empty and it becomes useless. These cells have a very short life so when they die, our bodies absorb the empty cast and won't replace them. With time, our bodies will extract the energy from food and give it to the organs that need them rather than storing them.

Because of this, the body will readjust and decrease the size and number of fat cells that will improve our metabolism, prolongs lives, treats disease, and decreases inflammation. If we keep this routine with time, our bodies will reabsorb the extra empty cells and will get rid of them as waste. This leaves us healthier and leaner on many levels.

Insulin

Whenever you consume a candy bar or meal, there is going to be glucose, fatty acids, or amino acids in the intestines that will tell the pancreas to secrete insulin. Insulin affects many different cells in the body, especially the fat tissues, liver, and muscles. Insulin will tell the cells to do:

- Begin building glycogen from glucose; fats from glycerol and fatty acids; and proteins from amino acids

- Quit breaking down fatty acids, glucose, and amino acids; proteins into amino acids; fats into fatty acids and glycerol; glycogen and glucose

- Absorb amino acids, fatty acids, and glucose

What the lipoprotein lipases do all depends on how much insulin is in the body. If there is a lot of insulin, then the lipases will become very active. If there isn't a lot of insulin in the body, then the lipases will become inactive.

The blood will absorb the fatty acids and then it will be sent to the liver, fat cells, and muscle. Within these cells, after being stimulated by the insulin, fatty acids are transformed into fat molecules which will be stored inside fat droplets.

Fat cells are able to take up glucose and amino acids that the blood has absorbed after you have eaten. They then convert these into fat molecules. Converting carbs or proteins into fat tends to be ten times less effective than simply storing extra fat into the fat cell, but the body isn't able to do it. If there are 100 extra calories of fat floating through the blood, the fat cells could only store it, and then use 2.5 calories for energy. If there are 100 extra glucose calories floating through your blood, your body will need 23 calories of energy in order to transform it from glucose into fat, and the rest is stored. If the fat cell had a choice, it would take hold of the fat and then store it instead of the carbs since fat is much easier to store.

How Our Bodies Break Down Fat

Whenever we go for a while without eating, the body won't absorb any food. If the body isn't absorbing food, there isn't much insulin in the blood. The body is constantly using energy and when our body isn't absorbing food, the energy we need has to come from our stores of fats, proteins, and carbs. When this is happening, the different organs will start to secrete hormones:

- Thyroid: thyroid hormone

- Adrenal gland: adrenaline

- Pituitary gland: adrenocorticotropic hormone

- Pituitary gland: growth hormone

- Pancreas: glucagon

These hormones act with the cells in fat tissue, muscles, and the liver and work in the opposite way that insulin does.

When you aren't eating, or if you are exercising, the body has to find its energy from other internal stores. The main source of energy will always be glucose. Some cells in the body, like the cells of the brain, only gets its energy from glucose.

The first thing the body does when trying to keep energy is to start breaking down glycogen or carbs to created glucose. This process is what is known as glycogenolysis. After this is used up, the body will start to break down fat into fatty acids and glycerol, which is called lipolysis. The body will then immediately break these fatty acids down for energy, or it can also be used to form glucose in the multi-step process called gluconeogenesis. During this process, amino acids will be used to create more glucose.

Inside the fat cells, different forms of lipases will breakdown the fats to create glycerol and fatty acids. The lipases will become activated by several different hormones like epinephrine, growth hormones, and glucagon. The fatty acids and glycerol that resulted are then released into the blood which will travel through to the liver and back out into the blood. When it gets into the liver, the fatty acids and glycerol could be either used to make glucose or broken down further.

• Losing Fat and Losing Weight

Your weight gets determined by how fast your body stores energy from what you eat and how quickly you use that energy. Keep in mind that as the body is breaking down fat, the number of fat cells is going to stay the same. The fat cells just become smaller.

Most experts are going to agree that one of the best options to maintain a good weight is to:

- Regularly exercise

- Don't eat in excess

- Consume a balanced diet

- Brown Fat: Makes Heat

With a newborn baby, their body doesn't have a lot of fat to help them retain body heat and insulate its body. While there is plenty of white fat, babies don't have any fat stored. The brown fat is smaller in size than the white fat and is full of small fat droplets. All of these have a bunch of mitochondria that generate a lot of heat. Newborn babies produce heat by turning fat molecules into fatty acids that are in the brown fat. Instead of those fatty acids leaving their cells, they are then broken down by the mitochondria and the body then releases the energy as heat. This is the same thing that happens in hibernating animals. These animals have extra brown fat. As a newborn starts to eat, they will start developing white fat and all of their brown fat will start to go away. Adults usually don't have much brown fat.

FASTING

Intermittent fasting has become a growing phenomenon over the last few years. It has had a strong impact on the dieting world. Its origins, however, are more ancient than most people realize. We are going to take a trip back in time to look at how fasting has played a part in the lives of humans for centuries.

Ancient Civilization

When the word fasting is said, it is hard for people not to picture a person starving to death. Fasting, though, isn't the same thing as starvation. Starvation isn't controlled or deliberate. People who are starving don't know when they will be getting their next meal. Fasting in primitive humans could be considered starvation since they didn't choose to go without food. It isn't the same as fasting today. In this day and age, fasting is completely voluntary.

Fasting has been around since the dawn of time. During primitive times, fasting wasn't a choice as much as a necessity. Fasting happened when it came to the availability and prevalence of food, and the hunter-gatherer's ability to acquire it.

During ancient times, people were forced to go for long periods of time between meals. This could go on for days depending on the availability of food. However, what came from this necessity was an incredible and sustainable emotional, mental, and physical effect.

As preservation techniques were found and knowledge of food grew, fasting didn't happen as often. They had food more readily available, but still, fasting continues to happen more often for many people. It probably wasn't until modern times that fasting became something that only certain religions followed and people had to do it when their doctors asked them to.

The ancient Greeks took their medical cues from nature. Humans, like most mammals, didn't eat when they were sick. Due to this, fasting is thought to be the "physician within." This instinct to fast is what makes cats, humans, and dogs anorexic when sick. This is something that I'm sure everyone has experienced. Think about the last time you had a stomach bug, a cold, or the flu. You probably couldn't even think about food. It seems like fasting is a universal human instinct to several different illnesses. This means that fasting is something that has been ingrained into humans.

Ancient Greeks thought fasting had the ability to improve cognitive abilities. Think back to the last big holiday where you gorged yourself. After, did you feel mentally alert and energetic, or did you feel dopey and sleepy? Chances are, you felt the latter. When you eat a lot, blood is sent to the digestive system in order to take care of the influx of food, leaving little blood to travel to the brain. This is what causes a food coma.

Religious Fasting

Part of the history of fasting is fasting for religious purposes. This type of fasting hasn't stopped. The only changes are some of the off-shoots of religions have changed their views slightly and removed fasting as part of their practices and rituals.

Buddhists also practice fasting. Nuns and monks follow the Vinaya rules, where they don't eat after the noon meal. They don't look at this as a fast. Rather, it is just a disciplined regimen that helps their health and meditation.

In Buddhist teachings, the Middle Path means they avoid extremes of indulgence and self-mortification. Prince Siddhartha, before attaining Buddahood, would practice short regimens of strict austerity that were followed by years of serenity meditation under the tutelage of two teachers in which he consumed minimal food. These austerities along with five other ascetics didn't improve his meditation, liberation, bring his closer to nirvana. After this, Prince Siddhartha would practice eating in moderation, which he advocated for his followers. However, lay Buddhists, on Uposatha days, had to observe the eight precepts which meant they abstained from food from noon until morning the next day.

There are many Christian denominations that practice fasting and it is often done on specific seasons of their calendar, or the fasting days are chosen by the individual's beliefs. The Lenten fast is observed by several Western Christianity denominations, including Western Orthodox Churches, Anglican Communion, Reformed Churches, Methodist Churches, Lutheran Churches, and the Catholic Church. The Lenten fast is a 40-day partial fast, this is meant to commemorate the fast that Christ observed while he was in the desert. While there are many who still observe the entire Lenten fast, Ash Wednesday and Good Friday tend to be emphasized as the normative days of fasting during this season.

Within the Roman Catholic faith, fasting is looked at as the reduction of the intake of food to just one meal. These meals aren't allowed to contain any meat on Good Friday, Ash Wednesday, and every Friday for the whole month unless a solemnity falls of a Friday. They also have two collations during the day, but they aren't allowed to equal a large meal. They can't eat solid foods between meals during fasts. People between the ages of 18 and 59 are required to fast. Abstaining from meat consumption is required on certain days by people over the age of 14. Meats don't include fish.

Pope Pius XII had relaxed a few of the regulations around fasting in 1956. Pope Paul VI, in 1966, created the Paenitemini and changed the fasting requirements for Roman Catholics. In his writing, it is recommended that fasting be appropriate for the economic situation of each Catholic and that fasting and abstaining be voluntary. Within the United States, the Roman Catholics only have two obligatory fasting days and they are Good Friday and Ash Wednesday.

Eastern Orthodox Christians look at fasting as a way to connect the body and soul and aren't seen as a purpose to suffer. Instead, they feel that fasting guards them against gluttony, as well as impure deeds, words, and thoughts. Fasting has to also include increased almsgiving and prayer. To fast without them is seen as useless or spiritually harmful. Their fasts typically last for 40 days during Lent, seven days during the Holy Week, 40 days during the Nativity Fast, eight to 42 days during the Apostles Fast, and for two weeks during the Dormition fast.

Fasting plays a huge part in the Hindu religion. People follow different fasts based on their personal beliefs and customs. Some will fast during certain days of the month, like Pradosha, Purnima, or Ekadasi. It all depends on their favorite deity. There are certain days of the week that are reserved for fasting. For example, people who follow Shiva will fast on Mondays. It is common in southern India for people to fast on Tuesday.

For Muslims, fasting doesn't include abstaining from food and drink. They also abstain from falsehoods in action and speech, indecent and ignorant speech, fighting, arguing, and having lustful thoughts. This means that fasting will strengthen their self-control.

During Ramadan, the believer's goal is to purify their soul and body and increase their good deeds. Overindulgence is avoided and they eat only enough to silence their hunger pains. Fasting for Ramadhan is obligatory for every Muslim. There are other non-obligatory fasts, which occur two days a week and during the middle of the moth. They are forbidden to fast on Eid al-Adha, Tashriw, and Eid al-Fitr.

Traditional Jewish practices observe fasts six days of the year. Besides Yom Kippur, fasting isn't permitted on Shabbat. The next major fasting day is Tisha B'Av. These are the two major fasts of the Jewish faiths. They observe their fasts from sunset to dusk the following day. The other four fasts they observe are viewed as minor and are optional and observed only from sun up to sundown. In the Ashkenazic tradition, the bride and groom customarily fast on their wedding before the ceremony because it represents their own personal Yom Kippur.

Fasting Today

Over the years, fasting has started to gain traction again outside of religious purposes. Intermittent fasting has spread wide and far now, and its impact on the health industry is growing. People have lost weight and seen energy improvements. The aging process has been slowed down and brain health has been improved.

Overall, intermittent fasting has been used throughout time for three purposes: body and mind health, spiritual connection, and survival. These are still valid today, but the focus is on the first, mind and body health. For people who want internal balance, intermittent fasting is the perfect solution.

Intermittent Fasting

What does intermittent fasting really mean today? A simple definition of intermittent fasting is restricting meals, cutting out eating days, or reducing the amount you snack. One of the more popular intermittent fasting schedules is the 5:2. With this schedule, you eat normally five days out of the week and you will fast the other two. There are other methods that focus on eating windows and fasting time throughout the day. The first thing that everyone should do is to cut out their snacking.

Many people have started snacking unconsciously or when they feel down. In fact, many people eat most of their meals unconsciously. They don't enjoy it and what it does for the body. They then end up confused as to why we are holding onto excess weight.

Intermittent fasting serves as a way to remind the body about the purpose of food. The great thing is, it is extremely simple to do. Cutting out a meal, reducing snacking, or just taking a day and consuming nothing but water is all you really have to do.

During the fasted state, the blood glucose levels will drop and cause a decrease in the production of insulin. If this happens, the body will send out a signal to begin burning fat for energy.

Intermittent fasting is a dietary and lifestyle choice, but those who end up being the most successful are those who accept it as a lifestyle almost immediately. There are many dieting plans that match up with intermittent fasting, but for many, intermittent fasting is the only change they make. The main point is to consume less food and to eat less often. The body and brain will respond quickly.

The majority of people will begin intermittent fasting because they want to lose some weight. Some only want to lose a couple of pounds they gained during the holidays, while others want to lose more.

On the other hand, some people decide to try intermittent fasting in order to reverse the signs of aging, heal the brain, and heal the heart.

Lastly, some will be intermittent fasting because they aren't happy with how their body is working for them in terms of athletics. Some people aren't really heavy, but rather hefty, and they would like to slim down in the right places and bulk up in others. For these people, intermittent fasting can help to repurpose lingering fat to be burned off or become muscle.

While people begin intermittent fasting for various reasons, they all stick with it for the same, which is that the benefits are incredible and undeniable. Regardless of your reasoning for beginning, you will stick with this new lifestyle because you will see a change in your body. You will stick with it because you will look at yourself as stronger in many areas of your life and you are going to learn new things about yourself.

Myths

Intermittent fasting, while having served our ancestors for millennia, is not free of misrepresentation. People have a lot of preconceived notions about intermittent fasting, and we are going to take a moment to bust these myths.

- Your body will hit starvation mode

Your body isn't going to enter starvation mode if you are following an intermittent fasting regimen. Going slightly longer between meals or skipping a meal or two isn't going to cause your body to think you are starving. It will help remind your body how to absorb important nutrients.

- You will lose muscle

This works a lot like the one above. Just like the body isn't going to hit starvation mode after you have skipped a meal, it won't cause your body to lose muscle mass. The only way you would start to lose muscle mass is if you were starving, but once again, you should not start starving when intermittent fasting. The only way either one of these could happen is if you overdo your fasting and go for too long without eating.

- You will overeat when you do eat, and this isn't healthy.

While many people will have an instinct to overeat during eating times, not everyone will. Even those who make the mistake of overeating when they first begin intermittent fasting will learn how to overcome this instinct. Your body will try to talk you into overeating at first since it doesn't realize what is happening, but if you keep your portion sizes normal and keep yourself from snacking, your body will adjust, as will your appetite.

- Your metabolism will slow down.

The truth is that your metabolism won't slow down because you don't eat as often. People who believe this to be true assume that restricted caloric intake will make their metabolism to slow over time, but intermittent fasting isn't as much about cutting caloric intake. It is more about cutting down the time at which the calories are consumed. You don't have to restrict your daily calorie intake. It all depends on you and what type of diet you choose to follow while fasting.

- You will gain weight if you begin skipping meals.

The same logic that created myth three is the same logic behind this myth. If you don't work through the urge to gorge yourself during your eating window, you will gain some weight but most people don't have this problem. Many people will realize they are gorging themselves and will stop since they won't be seeing the results they want. Skipping a meal never guarantees a person will gain weight. People who skip a meal and overeat will likely see some weight gain.

- When fasting, you can't eat anything.

This is a half-and-half myth. There is a little bit of truth to it. This only holds true for the intermittent fasting methods of 12:12, 14:10, 16:8, and 20:4.

These require fasting and eating every day. With these methods, there are going to be certain hours each day where you aren't supposed to eat anything. The same doesn't hold true for methods that have days on and days off. With these methods, the fasting period doesn't keep you from eating. Instead, you will only eat fewer calories. With methods like 5:2 or eat-stop-eat, you are allowed to consume up to 500 calories on your fasting days.

- There is only one way to intermittent fast that will actually work.

This is so false, it's funny. There isn't a single way to practice intermittent fasting, and the main reason why intermittent fasting is so popular is that there are so many different methods. Everyone has different bodies and personality types and they are going to be drawn to different methods. Intermittent fasting is about self-correction, flexibility, and adjustments. No single method is going to work for everyone. That is why you can pick whichever method that works best for you.

- It isn't natural to fast.

We have already busted this myth. Fasting is more natural than it is to shove food in your mouth when you are not hungry. Fasting has a deep connection to our evolution. It helps our digestive system, cells, heart, and brain to give ourselves a break from food. The only thing that makes intermittent fasting seems wrong is myths like these.

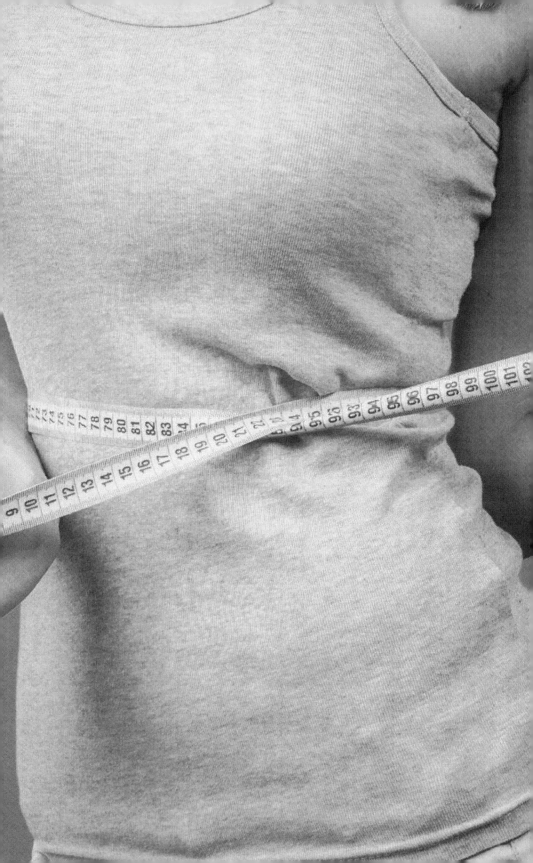

INTERMITTENT FASTING TYPES

There are lots of different methods of intermittent fasting that you can pick from so that it works for your life. All of these different methods have one main purpose, alternating between a fed and fasted stated.

There are nine main methods for intermittent fasting that we will discuss in this chapter. We will talk through the pros and cons of each of these, and I will help you to figure out how to pick one. Having these different plans should help to ease your apprehension around intermittent fasting because you will have the option of choosing the one that works for you.

I feel as if there are some people who believe that intermittent fasting has only one schedule that everybody must follow. Most diets are like that. If you want a diet to work, you don't have the option to pick and choose what works for you. Intermittent fasting doesn't work that you. That's why it is so important that you do your research.

Lean-Gains

This first type of fasting schedule focuses on a combination of a healthy diet, fasting, and rigorous exercise. This is what bodybuilders will typically choose because it helps in muscle building. The main goal of this is to fast for 14 to 16 hours each day. The fast starts at the end of your last meal and lasts until your first meal the next day, normally around noon or 1 o'clock.

With this schedule, people will exercise an hour before their first meal. They can do whatever exercise they want to do. When they have their first meal, it will be their largest in order to help their muscles recover.

After that first meal, the rest of the day will go on as normal. There are some who will still try to eat three meals in the shortened eating window, eating at 4 and then 9. Others will just have two meals. When beginning, you don't have to go a full 15 hours for your fast. You can begin with a shorter fasting window and slowly make it bigger until you reach the number of hours you want.

Lean-Gains is better suited for bodybuilders and people who want to gain muscles.

16/8 Method

This is probably the most popular intermittent fasting schedule. This will look similar to the Lean-Gains method, but this method doesn't emphasize a workout regimen. Essentially, all you have to do is fast for a total of 16 hours each day and then eat during the other eight. Most people will choose to place their eight-hour eating window during the time of the day where they are most active. That means if you tend to be more active during the night, you can wait until later in the day to have your first meal. Some people will eat from 3 to 11, while others may eat from 11 to 7.

This is a very flexible schedule, and this is one that works for the majority of people. If you find that eating during a certain time isn't working, then you change it the next day. The best part is that the majority of your fasting time is going to happen while you are sleeping. To make things even easier, make sure you time your waking fasted hours to be during a period where you don't have the time to think about food.

If you have a lot going on first thing in the morning, then finish up your fasted hours then and eat around noon or one. If you have a slow morning, then eat around nine or ten, and start fasting in the afternoon. You can pick whatever works best.

Lean-gains tend to be stricter in the timing and won't give you as much flexibility as this method. Lean-gains requires having a strict diet and exercise regimen as well, whereas this method does not. It is smart, though, to make sure you eat sensible foods during your eating windows. This will ensure you see better results. You don't have to count calories, though. People experience more side effects from fasting when they start counting calories because they don't eat enough.

14/10 Method

This method works exactly like the last method except you have a longer eating period and a shorter fasting period. You will only fast for 14 hours, and then eat during the other ten. This is a good place to start for people who want to ease into the above method or any of the other methods we will talk about. It won't seem as hard.

12/12 Method

This works like the previous two, except you fast and eat for an equal amount of hours. This is a bit easier than the last method. It is a good idea to make sure that you set cut-offs for this method because it is very easy to end up eating too early or too late.

20/4 Method

This one is harder than the previous methods because of the longer fasting window. You will be fasting for the majority of the day and will like only have one large meal, or several small snacks. You should definitely not start with this method. Like the previous ones, the eating and fasted windows are adjustable.

This one can be tricky because people will either over-eat or under-eat during their eating window. Neither is a good idea nor do you have to. When you do eat, make sure that you keep your portions at a normal size. This is why it might be smarter to do smaller snack type meals during the four-hour window instead of trying to get your caloric needs all in one meal.

If this method turns out to be too hard for you, then step it back to the 16/8 method.

5/2 Method

This works very well for people who have an all-or-nothing attitude. You don't have to fast and eat every single day with this one. Instead, you have two days where you fast the whole day. The other five days you will eat and exercise as you normally would. The fasting days are strict, so you don't want them to be consecutive.

Now, you don't go without food completely on those fasting days. You get to eat only 500 calories on those days. So, I supposed you could call them "restricted-intake" days.

This is probably one of the harder methods to follow, even though you often have great weight loss results on this one. It also means that it is a lot easier to over eat the day after a restricted day, so you have to make sure that your willpower is strong. It may be a good idea to start with a 16/8 method to get used to fasting before going into the 5/2 method.

The Warrior Method

This will seem similar to the 20/4 method we already talked about because it requires a 20 hour fast every day. The difference is the mindset and outlook. The thought process behind this method is during ancient times, hunters would return home from hunting or the warrior came back from battle to only a meal every day. That meal had to be what provided them with the energy and nutrients to survive the rest of the day.

So, people who follow this one are encouraged to have one large meal each day. This meal has to be loaded with carbs, proteins, and fats so that they can make it through the other 20 hours.

This is often too intense for most people. If this doesn't feel right for you after a day or two, don't force yourself to continue. If you can, try to make it through a week. Otherwise, go to a method that is a bit easier.

Alternate Day Method

This is close to the 5/2 method and the next method. It focuses on days on and days off of eating and fasting. The biggest difference is that for this one, you will normally start with two fasting days, but you can build it up to four.

Some people will become very strict with this method and will fast every other day, which means eating no more than 500 calories on the fasting days. Some people do this in a more flexible fashion and will have two regular days followed by one fasting day. You can pick what is best for you.

You can either make this harder or easier than the 5/2 method. Surprisingly, people who have an intense workout schedule will find that the more intense this method is, the better it works for them. Those who consume more than 2000 calories on feeding days have more gains.

Eat/Stop/Eat

This is sometimes referred to as the 24-hour method. This is like the last method but is less intense and more flexible. For this one, on your fast days, you don't have to worry about eating 500 calories. You pick how many days each week you fast, but there has to be at least one feeding day between your fast days. If you only want one fast day a week, then so be it.

The best way to approach this method is to make sure you have a strict diet or are choosing to eat healthy foods during the feeding times. To see success with this, you are going to have to have some type of calorie restriction.

On your fasting days, you have the choice of either eating up to 500 calories or not eating anything at all. But, please, make sure that you drink lots of water. Allowing yourself to become dehydrated is one of the worst things that you can do when you are fasting.

If you plan on working out, you need to make sure that you only work out on the days you eat. This is true also for the 5/2 method. If you do any type of workout on fasting days, make sure that it is some light like stretching or yoga.

Spontaneous Fasting

While most of these methods are very flexible, this is the most flexible of them all. This method only requires you to skip a meal or two during your day whenever you want or when your body feels it's right.

This is a pretty good option for people who have a sensitive digestive system or a set fitness schedule. This also tends to work well for people who have a very hectic schedule and those who find that they need a little more energy at different times of the day.

Despite the fact that this could be chaotic and unorganized, this method can end up being very structured. There are some people who will choose the meals that they skip every day instead of just skipping whenever. This method is meant to help people make fasting work no matter what their life looks like.

Choosing the Best Method

There are many different things to think about when you are picking your IF method. One of the most important things to remember is that you have the power to change your method if your first choice isn't working for you. You can also troubleshoot all of the methods as well.

The main things that you need to think about when you are choosing your method are:

- Dietary Choices – Are you looking to change your diet? Are you already consuming a healthy diet? Do you like counting calories? How much processed foods do you eat? What you choose to eat will play a big part in your method. If you don't mind counting calories, then 5/2, alternate-day, or eat/stop/eat could work for you. Fasting every day could work for those who haven't quite adopted a healthy eating habit.

- Family and Friends – Do the people around you follow a healthy diet? Do they like to share their opinions? Do you have a support system or do they make fun of you? This might not seem like something that is important, but how people treat you based on your health choices will dictate whether you succeed or fail. Some people may think what you are doing is stupid or going to hurt you, so you need to make sure you are mentally prepared for what they are going to say or what you will tell them. You may soon find that there are toxic people in your life that you need to cut out. Hopefully, though, you will have just as many who will lift you up and help you.

- Work – Are you allowed to freely eat at work? Is there a lot of food at your place of work? Do you stand a lot or do strenuous activities? You want to ensure that you will have the energy to do your job, so if you move around a lot or do strenuous things at work, fasting while you work probably isn't a good idea. Otherwise, fasting at work may be the best time because your mind will be distracted.

- Daily Tendencies – What do you normally eat? When do you work? Is your daily routine flexible? Is there a lot of travel involved in your life? Do you move a lot? Do you have a hard time remembering when to eat? Do you work out regularly? You need to think about every little thing in your daily life when it comes to picking your method. Does it make sense for you to have days where you greatly restrict your calories?

Pick a method that makes sense for your habits.

- Lifestyle – When do you get up? How long do you sleep? How hungry are you when you get up? What is your job? Do you spend most of your day in a car, at a desk, or on your feet? Do you spend most of your day alone or around lots of other people? When you start picking your method, think about the different aspects of your lifestyle. It would be best to not choose a method where you aren't allowed to eat when you will need the most energy. Most methods are flexible, so you can probably adjust them to work with your needs after you get started.

- Body Type and Abilities – Take a moment to think about how you look and feel in the present and what you are looking to change. Think about the way your body reacts to food and how you feel when you become hungry. Think about what you think your limits are and how much you want to push them. Do you sit on the couch most of the day, or are you always on the move? Is your body type slim or not? Does your body like to hold onto fit or do you build muscle quickly? Do you retain water? Compare this to your goals and choose the method that will do the most for you to reach those goals.

Above all else, make sure you do what feels right to you. You need to fully and completely understand what your goals are for fasting. If at any point you start to feel like you are sacrificing your health to reach those goals, start troubleshooting and adjusting your method. Your body could be letting you know that you need to stop.

The first method you choose may not be the best choice for you, so don't feel discouraged if you discover that you need to change things up.

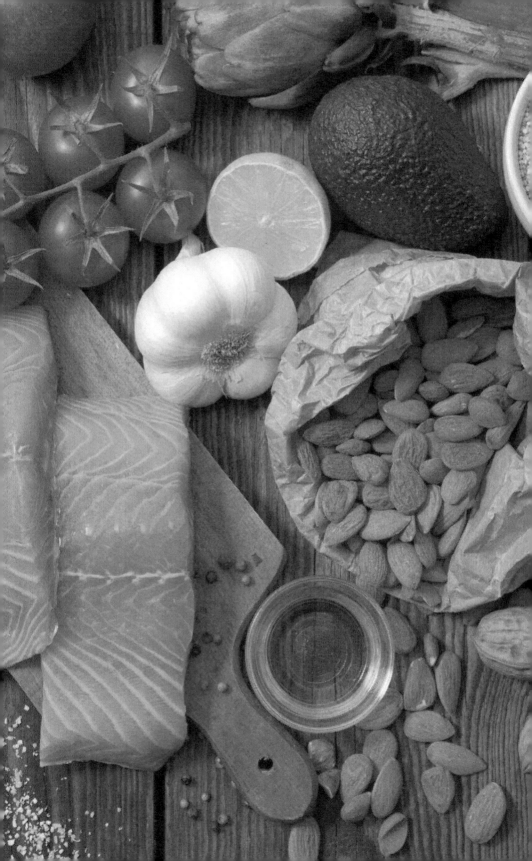

INTERMITTENT FASTING AND KETO

The ketogenic diet and intermittent fasting are two different weight-loss strategies that have a lot of similarities. In both instances, ketones are produced and the body will burn more fat. If you put them together, they become a very powerful duo.

A lot of people will use these two strategies together to bust through plateaus, increase weight loss, and improve energy. Some people will even use this combination to help with durability.

In this chapter, we are going to go over how keto and intermittent fasting can be used together to reach your weight loss goals and to improve your health.

What Is Keto?

In the simplest of terms, a ketogenic diet is a very low-carb, high-fat diet. This isn't some new diet, either. It was first created in the 1920s as a treatment for children who suffered from epilepsy. Studies have found that a low-carb high-fat diet will increase a person's ketone levels, and when the brain has to run off of ketones, they people didn't have as many seizures. This is still used today, but there has been more investigation to see if it is a breakthrough treatment for several other diseases and neurological disorders. So, this isn't just some weight loss trend.

The main purpose of this diet is to place the body into ketosis. The body burns carbs as energy. But if the amount of carbs in the body is restricted, the body will start breaking down the fat stored within the body, and this will create what is known as ketones. These ketones are then used as fuel.

The biggest benefit of following a ketogenic diet is weight loss, but there are many other benefits that come along with it, such as:

- Control of diabetes
- Hormonal balance
- Improvement in epilepsy
- Mental clarity
- Appetite suppression
- Improvement in migraines
- Reduces cholesterol
- Prevents cancer

Move from the 1920s, researchers started to find that the keto diet provided benefits other than the control of epilepsy. Many wellness professionals, the world over, are embracing the word ketogenic. Many people have started using this diet to control and prevent diabetes and to lose weight.

Many studies have found that the ketogenic diet, as well as other low-carb diets, are perfect for losing weight. They tend to work better than a low-fat or reduced-calorie diet. The ketogenic diet is sometimes easier to follow because ketones can work as an appetite suppressant. Without consuming a lot of carbohydrates, you aren't faced with sugar crashes or cravings for carbs. You just eat plenty of fat to keep you feeling full.

What Are Ketones?

Your metabolism can create three different types of ketones:

- Acetate – Acetone

- Beta-hydroxybutyrate – BHB

- Acetoacetate – AcAc

The two main ketones that get produced are BHB and AcAc. Acetate is one of the least abundant ketones. Your blood always contains some level of ketones, but these levels will increase when you fast, exercise, and sleep. When fasting overnight, around two and six percent of your energy is supplied by ketones.

Ketone levels may increase so high that they are in control of 50% of your energy and 70% of the brain's energy. This is what we call ketosis, and this can only happen if you greatly reduce your carb intake and keep your protein intake at a minimum. Eating fewer than 50 grams, typically around 20 grams, of crabs and 60 grams of protein will place your body into ketosis.

There are also synthetic ketones on the market known as exogenous ketones. These can help you to get into a state of ketosis faster than with dieting alone.

- How do you form ketones?

The body normally needs glucose for energy. Glucose is found in proteins and carbs. Your body prefers glucose as fuel because it is much easier to change it into energy and it can easily be stored for later use. The problem is, glucose dissolves fat, and when this happens, it is releases free radicals that are harmful to you.

If you limit your carb intake for a single day, your body will need the glucose that has been stored in the muscles and liver. This is what is referred to as glycogen. The liver has enough glycogen stored to work the brain for about 12 hours if no more carbs are consumed. Once those 12 hours have passed, the body will turn to burn stored fat, which is the best energy reserve your body has. When you limit the carbs you eat and consume plenty of healthy fats, your body will continue to use fats for energy.

One the best thing about having a body deprived of carbs is that after 24 to 48 hours, the liver will start changing fatty acids into ketone bodies. This whole process is referred to as ketogenesis and it is the big metabolic switch that all keto followers want to happen.

What Are the Benefits?

People can choose to enter ketosis for several different reasons. One of the main reasons is to lose weight, but there are other reasons like controlling blood sugar, better mental clarity, lower risk of cancer, and more energy.

There was a time when researchers viewed ketones as something that was bad or toxic. As more studies have been done, it was discovered that there are a lot of misconceptions about them and that ketones are actually good for you.

The following are just a few of the benefits of ketones:

- Weight Loss – The body has to burn fat to make ketones. When this happens, natural ketosis is going to cause weight loss. There are some studies that suggest ketones can help you lose weight while also curbing your appetite.

- Diabetes Control – Many low-carb diets, like the keto diet, have been found to do a great job at lowering blood sugar levels and insulin resistance. There are studies that have found that BHB ketone can reduce inflammation which is another way to control diabetes.

- Longevity – If you want to stay healthy and live a long life, occasionally fasting can help you do that. Studies have found that restricting carbs can help to lengthen your life expectancy.

- Preventing Cancer – Glucose can increase cancer cells. When you don't let them have their favorite food, it can help to reduce cancer cells and may help prevent and treat cancer. Many people who are at risk of developing cancer or who are being treated for cancer will follow a ketogenic diet.

- Resilience – Ketone bodies can provide your body with powerful and constant energy. They can also help to preserve your performance and resilience better than glucose ever could.

- Brainpower – The ketogenic diet was originally meant to be an epilepsy treatment, but it has been found as a great way to protect the neurons in the brain. It can improve focus, mental energy, and create a sharper mind.

Fasting and a keto diet can help to improve your overall health by balanced blood glucose, improving your defense from free radicals, and reducing inflammation.

Common Side Effects of Keto

A ketogenic diet will sometimes cause side effects for people. When you first start out, you may experience what is known as the keto flu. This will feel a lot like the regular flu in that you feel nauseous, tired, and may have headaches. This is the real flu and will pass once your body gets adapted to using ketones as fuel. That being said, if the ketogenic diet is something that you want to try, you may want to start off with an intermittent fasting protocol first without any dietary changes. After a month or so of fasting, you can ease into a keto diet and you may not experience as many side effects.

Fasting and Keto Together

You know all of the different ways to fast, and you know what the ketogenic diet is. The main purpose of intermittent fasting is to not eat as much during the day. Intermittent fasting has the ability to boost your fat burning. When your body is a fasted state, your body will turn to your fat stores for energy. This is when the body starts forming ketones to fuel you and your brain. Now, the ketogenic diet does the same thing without any fasting. But, something that a lot of people will find when following a keto diet is that they don't feel as hungry. This means that they start fasting simply because they don't feel like they need to eat.

You don't have to fast when on keto, and you don't have to follow keto when fasting. You can choose to do one or the other, but some people will find that fasting becomes easier on a ketogenic diet.

People who follow a ketogenic diet will have lower insulin levels and blood glucose levels. They have a reduced appetite because of the effects of the ketogenic diet. This means that they won't have any sugar crashes, and they won't feel as hungry.

If you maintain a regular diet, high in carbs, and you fast, you may experience an increase in hunger hormones and your blood glucose may drop quickly. This could end up causing you to feel irritable, shaky, and weak. It could mean that you feel hungry all of the time. This doesn't always happen, though.

Using the ketogenic diet and intermittent fasting for weight loss is a great idea, but just remember, you can use them separately as well.

FOODS, DRINKS, RECIPES

When it comes to intermittent fasting, there aren't any restrictions or specifications about the foods you eat or how much you eat during your feeding time. But, you probably aren't going to see a lot of weight loss if you are constantly eating Reese Cups.

To get the most out of your fasting, you want to aim for a well-balanced diet during the feeding times in order to lose weight, maintain your energy, and to stick to your diet. You need to turn to foods like lean proteins, dairy, seeds, beans, nuts, whole grains, veggies, and fruits.

Choosing high-fiber and unprocessed, whole foods will serve you the most when it comes to losing weight. Here are some foods that you should make sure you eat plenty of.

1. Water

Even when you aren't eating, you need to make sure that you stay hydrated. Hydration keeps all of your major organs working properly. How much water you should drink depends on your body, but you should aim to have your urine pale yellow in color. If your urine is dark, that means you are dehydrated, which can also make you feel lightheaded, fatigued, and cause headaches. If you couple that with lower food intake, it can be a recipe for disaster. If you don't like plain water, try adding some mint leaves, lemon juice, or cucumber to the water.

2. Avocados

While this may be a high caloric food, its monounsaturated fats are extremely satiating. One study has found that having half of one with your lunch can help you to feel fuller for longer.

3. Fish

There are lots of reasons to try and consume eight ounces of fish each week. It is full of protein and healthy fats, and it contains plenty of vitamin D. Fish is called "brain food."

4. Cruciferous Veggies

These are foods like cauliflower, broccoli, and Brussels sprouts, and they are full of fiber. When you are limiting the amount of food you eat during the day, fiber-rich foods can help to keep you going and prevents constipation.

5. Potatoes

Not every single white food is bad. There have been studies performed that have found that potatoes are one of the most satiating foods. Another study discovered that consuming potatoes as part of a balanced diet can help you to lose weight. Potato chips and fried don't count, though.

6. Legumes and Beans

These foods help to provide you with energy. These are carb-heavy, so you don't want to overdo them, but they are a great part of a well-balanced diet. Plus, foods like lentils, peas, black beans, and chickpeas have been found to help lower body weight, even when there isn't any calorie restriction.

7. Probiotics

You've got to keep those critters in your gut happy. They need probiotics, and you can get those in foods like kraut, kombucha, or kefir. There are also supplements you can take to help keep your gut healthy.

8. Berries

Berries have lots of vitamins and nutrients. Strawberries, specifically, have more than 100% of the daily value of vitamin C in a single cup. Plus, berries are rich in flavonoids, and one study found people who consumed a lot of flavonoids had a smaller BMI increase over a 14-year span than people who didn't.

9. Eggs

One egg has six grams of protein and it doesn't take that long to cook. Making sure you get plenty of protein will ensure that you don't end up feeling hungry. A great snack is a hard-boiled egg.

10. Nuts

They may have more calories, but they also have healthy fats. The polyunsaturated fats in walnuts have the ability to change physiological markers for satiety and hunger.

11. Whole Grains

Many people are afraid of carbs nowadays, but they aren't necessarily bad. They have lots of fiber and healthy nutrients in them, and as long as you choose whole, and not refined, grains, they can help you to lose weight.

Now that you know what types of foods you should aim to consume. Here are some delicious recipes that you can try out.

Peachy Oatmeal

What you need:

- Pinch salt
- Cinnamon, .25 tsp
- Quick-cooking oats, .5 c
- Brown sugar, 2 tbsp
- Milk, .5 c
- Sliced peaches, .5 15-oz can
- Water, .5 c

What you will do:

1. Mix everything together in a microwavable bowl. Cook for a minute on high. Stir, and cook for another minute. Do this until the oats have softened up.

Egg White Omelet

What you need:

- Egg white substitute, 32 oz
- Pepper
- Chopped mushrooms, 2 tbsp
- Salt
- Chopped green bell pepper, 2 tbsp
- Chopped onion, 2 tbsp

What you will do:

1. Using a glass loaf pan, spray it with some cooking spray, and then add in the mushrooms, bell pepper, and onion. Sprinkle in some pepper and salt and then add in the egg whites.

2. Place in the microwave and cook for three minutes. Take it out and stir the mixture. Microwave another three minutes. If it still runny, cook in 30-second intervals until cooked through. Sprinkle with more pepper and salt if needed.

Apple Pie Smoothie

What you need:

- Dash of nutmeg
- Cinnamon, 1 tsp
- Apple juice, 2 c
- Chopped banana
- Pumpkin pie filling, .5 c
- Vanilla yogurt, 2 6-oz containers

What you will do:

1. Add all of the above ingredients into a blender and mix until smooth.

Morning Shot of Vitamin C

What you need:

- Honey, 1 tbsp
- Orange juice, 1 c
- Vanilla yogurt, 1 c
- Large orange
- Frozen banana
- Nectarines, 2

What you will do:

1. Add all of the above ingredients into your blender and mix until it becomes smooth.

Wake Me Up Smoothie

What you need:

- Vanilla, 1 tsp
- Wheat germ, .25 c
- Strawberries, 1 c
- Vanilla yogurt, 2 c
- Bananas, 1
- Pineapple juice, 2 c

What you will do:

1. Add all of the above ingredients into your blender and mix until smooth.

Berry Parfait

What you need:

- Pinch of nutmeg
- Crushed graham crackers, 2 tbsp
- Frozen mixed berries, 10 oz
- Vanilla yogurt, 2 8-oz containers

What you will do:

1. In two glasses, add a layer of yogurt to each. Sprinkle in some berries. Continue doing this until the glasses are full, making sure the top layer is fruit. Top with the nutmeg and graham crackers.

Breakfast Brownies

What you need:

- Mashed banana
- Salt, .25 tsp
- Cinnamon, .5 tsp
- Baking powder, 1 tsp
- Quick-cooking oats, 1.5 c
- Flaxseed meal, .75 c
- Brown sugar, .75 c
- All-purpose flour, .5 c
- Vanilla, 1 tsp
- Egg
- Rice milk, .25 c

What you will do:

1. Start by setting your oven to 350. Grease an eight by ten casserole dish.

2. Stir together the salt, cinnamon, baking powder, brown sugar, oats, flour, and flaxseed meals. In another bowl, stirs the vanilla, egg, rice milk, and banana together. Add this into the flour mixture. Stir everything together and then add it to the casserole dish.

3. Bake for 20 minutes. Cover the pan with a towel and let it sit for five minutes. Slice and serve.

Chocolate Chip Oatmeal Pancakes

What you need:

- Soy milk, 1.5 c
- Vegan carob chips, .25 c
- Ground flaxseeds, .25 c
- Sea salt, .5 tsp
- Baking soda, .5 tsp
- Rolled oats, .75 c
- Baking powder, 2 tsp
- Flour, .75 c

What you will do:

1. Grease up a skillet and let it heat up as you mix everything together.

2. Mix everything together, except for the soy milk. Slowly add the soy milk in until everything comes together.

3. Add ¼ cup of the batter to the pan. Cook for a couple of minutes or until bubbles start to form and then flip and cook for a couple of minutes more.

Quinoa Porridge

What you need:

- Salt
- Vanilla, 1 tsp
- Brown sugar, 2 tbsp
- Water, .5 c
- Almond milk, 1.5 c
- Cinnamon, .25

What you will do:

1. Add the quinoa to a pot and add in the cinnamon. Cook for about three minutes, or until toasted, stirring often. Add in the vanilla, water, and milk. Then mix in the salt and sugar. Let everything come to a boil, cooking for about 25 minutes or until everything is thickened and cooked. You can add extra water if you need to.

Summery Fruit Parfait

What you need:

- Granola, .33 c
- Sliced banana, .5
- Wheat germ, 1 tbsp
- Vanilla yogurt, 6 oz
- Blueberries, .75 c
- Sliced strawberries, .75 c

What you will do:

1. In a cup, add a third of the strawberries, a third of the blueberries, a third of the yogurt, a third of the wheat germ, a third of the banana, and two tablespoons of the granola. Repeat this until you have added all of the ingredients.

Fava Bean Breakfast

What you need:

- Chopped parsley, .25 c
- Cumin, 1 tsp
- Diced tomato
- Chopped onion
- Olive oil, 1.5 tbsp
- Fava beans, 15 oz
- Red pepper flakes
- Pepper
- Salt
- Lemon juice, .25 c

What you will do:

1. Add the beans to a pot and let it come up to a boil. Stir in all of the other ingredients. Let everything come to a boil again and then let it simmer for five minutes. Serve this with a grilled pita.

Watermelon Salad

What you need:

- Lime zest, 2 tbsp
- Lemon zest, 2 tbsp
- Halved red grapes, 4 c
- Chopped watermelon, 4 c

What you will do:

1. Toss everything together and let it chill for an hour before serving.

Mango Breakfast Smoothie

What you need:

- Oats, .25 c
- Orange juice, .5 c
- Plain yogurt, .33 c
- Diced banana, .5
- Frozen mango chunks, .5 c

What you will do:

1. Add all of the smoothie ingredients into your blender and then mix them together until smooth.

Grapefruit Berry Smoothie

What you need:

- Crushed ice, 1 c
- Fresh grapefruit juice, 1.33 c
- Honey, 2 tbsp
- Strawberry banana yogurt, 8 oz
- Strawberries, 8
- Sliced bananas, 2

What you will do:

1. Add all of the smoothie ingredients into your blender and mix together until it becomes smooth. You may want to wait on adding the ice. You may not need it.

Superfood Breakfast

What you need:

- Honey, .5 tsp
- Dried goji berries, 2 tbsp
- Cinnamon, .5 tsp
- Ground almonds, 1 tbsp
- Blueberries, .25 c
- Unsweetened cocoa powder, 1 tsp
- Ground walnuts, 1 tbsp
- Ground flaxseed, 1 tbsp
- Nonfat plain yogurt, 1 c

What you will do:

1. Add everything into a bowl and mix it all together so that everything is well coated in the yogurt and the cocoa powder is mixed in.

Power Protein Smoothie

What you need:

- Dates, 2
- Bananas, 2
- Ground flaxseeds, 3 tbsp
- Water, .5 c
- Kale leaves, 5
- Almond milk, .5 c
- Frozen blueberries, 1.5 c

What you will do:

1. Place all of the above ingredients into a blender and mix them all together until they are smooth.

Hot Cereal

What you need:

- Amaranth, .5 c
- Cornmeal, .5 c
- Flaxseeds, .5 c
- Brown basmati rice, 1 c
- Sesame seeds, .5 c
- Quinoa, .5 c
- Buckwheat groats, .5 c
- Millet, .5 c

What you will do:

1. Place the rice into a coffee grinder and mix until it makes a coarse powder. Place this into a bowl. Do the same thing with the flaxseeds, sesame seeds, buckwheat, millet, and quinoa. Then mix in the amaranth and cornmeal. When you want to cook some, boil four cups of water with a bit of salt. Add in a cup of the mixture and let it simmer for 20 minutes.

Strawberry Smoothie

What you need:

- Sugar, 1.5 tsp
- Soy milk, 1 c
- Vanilla extract, .5 tsp
- Frozen strawberries, 14
- Chopped banana
- Rolled oats, .5 c

What you will do:

1. Add all of the above ingredients into your blender and then mix them together until they are smooth.

Whole Wheat Pancakes

What you need:

- Blueberries, .5 c
- Stevia, 1 tbsp
- Salt, .5 tsp
- Milk, 1 c
- Egg
- Baking powder, 2 tsp
- Whole wheat flour, 1.25 c

What you will do:

1. Sift the baking powder and flour together and set to the side. Whisk together the stevia, salt, milk, and egg. Mix in the flour mixture, stirring until everything just comes together. Fold in the blueberries.

2. Heat up a pan and coat it with some oil. Add ¼ cup of the batter into the heated pan. Cook on the first side until it starts to form bubbles. Flip and cook for a few more minutes on the other side. Continue cooking until you have used all of the batters.

Blueberry Muffins

What you need:

- Salt, .25 tsp
- Baking soda, 1 tsp
- Wheat germ, .25 c
- Quick-cooking oats, .25 c
- Baking powder, 1 tsp
- Oat bran, .25 c
- Sugar, .75 c
- All-purpose flour, .75 c
- Blueberries, 1 c
- Whole wheat flour, .75 c
- Vanilla, 1 tsp
- Vegetable oil, 1 tbsp
- Egg
- Buttermilk, 1 c
- Mashed banana
- Chopped walnuts, .5 c

What you will do:

1. Start by setting your oven to 350. Add paper liners to a 12-cup muffin tin.

2. Mix the salt, both flours, baking soda, sugar, baking powder, oats, oat bran, and wheat germ together. Stir in the walnuts and blueberries. In another bowl, stir the vanilla, oil, egg, buttermilk, and banana together. Add the banana mixture to the flour mixture and mix everything together. Divide this between the muffin cups.

3. Bake these for about 15 to 18 minutes. The tops should bounce back when pressed lightly. Enjoy.

Green Smoothie

What you need:

- Spinach, 1.5 c
- Chopped apple, .5
- Vanilla yogurt, 6 oz
- Grapes, 1 c
- Chopped banana

What you will do:

1. Place all of the above ingredients into a blender and mix until smooth. You may need to scrape the sides down from time to time.

Banana and Kale Smoothie

What you need:

- Maple syrup, 1 tsp
- Flaxseeds, 1 tbsp
- Unsweetened soy milk, .5 c
- Chopped kale, 2 c
- Banana

What you will do:

1. Add all of the above ingredients into a blender and mix until it forms a smooth drink.

Brighten Your Day Smoothie

What you need:

- Vanilla nonfat yogurt, 1 c
- Orange juice, 1 c
- Chopped banana
- Diced, peeled and seeded mango

What you will do:

1. Add all of the above ingredients into a blender and mix everything together until it becomes smooth.

Purple Smoothie

What you need:

- Vanilla, 1 tsp
- Honey, 1 tbsp
- Orange juice, 1 c
- Frozen blueberries, .5 c
- Frozen bananas, 2

What you will do:

1. Add in the fruit to a blender and mix until smooth. Mix in the vanilla and honey to your taste. You can add extra juice if it is too thick.

Applesauce Muffins

What you need:

- Egg
- Baking powder, 1 tsp
- Applesauce, .5 c
- Brown sugar, .5 c
- Buttermilk, 1 c
- Baking soda, .5 tsp
- Rolled oats, 1 c
- Whole wheat flour, 1 c

What you will do:

1. Add the oats into a bowl and then pour in the buttermilk. Let the oats rest for at least two hours at room temp.

2. Next, heat up your oven to 375 and line a 12-cup muffin with liners. Mix together the sugar, flour, baking powder, and baking soda. Slowly add in the oat mixture, along with the egg and applesauce. Divide into the muffin cups.

3. Place the muffins in the oven and cook for 30 minutes.

Coconut Oatmeal

What you need:

- Dried cranberries, .33 c
- Maple syrup, .25 c
- Rolled oats, 2 c
- Salt, .25 tsp
- Plain soy milk, 3.5 c
- Honey, 3 tbsp
- Plain yogurt, 8 oz
- Chopped walnuts, .33 c
- Sweetened coconut flakes, .33 c

What you will do:

1. Add the salt and milk to a pot and let it come to a boil. Mix in the cranberries, raisins, maple syrup, and oats. Let this come back up to a boil and then turn it down. Allow it to simmer for five minutes. Mix in the coconut and walnuts, and then let it rest until it comes to your desired thickness. Spoon into bowls and serve with the honey and yogurt if you want.

Potato Cakes

What you need:

- Pepper
- All-purpose flour, 3 tbsp
- Salt
- Chopped onion
- Beaten eggs, 2
- Shredded and peeled potatoes, 5
- Vegetable oil, 3 tbsp

What you will do:

1. Mix the pepper, flour, onion, salt, eggs, and potatoes together.
2. Heat the oil in a skillet and drop a large spoonful of the potatoes onto the pan. Flatten it out into a pancake shape. Let it cook for about four minutes on both sides, or until browned. Enjoy.

Pumpkin Oatmeal

What you need:

- Cinnamon sugar, 1 tsp
- Pumpkin pie spice, .25 tsp
- Pumpkin puree, .5 c
- Milk, .75 c
- Quick-cooking oats, 1 c

What you will do:

1. Stir all of the ingredients together in a microwavable bowl. Microwave for a couple of minutes, stirring halfway through the cooking time. You can add more milk if you need to. Mix in the cinnamon sugar, pumpkin, and the spice blend.

Cinnamon Apple Oatmeal

What you need:

- Milk, 1 c
- Cinnamon, 1 tsp
- Rolled oats, .66 c
- Chopped apple
- Apple juice, .25 c
- Water, 1 c

What you will do:

1. Mix the apples, juice, and water together in a pot. Let this come up to a boil and then mix in the cinnamon and oats. Let it come back up to a boil and then turn the heat down. Let it cook for about three minutes, or until thickened to your liking. Serve and enjoy.

Banana Waffles

What you need:

- Sliced banana, 2
- Egg
- All-purpose flour, 1.25 c
- 1% milk, 1 c
- Nutmeg, pinch
- Salt, .5 tsp
- Baking powder, 3 tsp

What you will do:

1. Begin by heating up your waffle iron. Stir together the nutmeg, flour, salt, and baking powder. Mix in the eggs and milk until everything is smooth.

2. Grease your waffle iron and add two tablespoons of the batter onto the iron. Add a couple of slices of the banana on top and then pour on a couple more tablespoonfuls of batter. Close the lid and let it cook according to your waffle iron. Continue until all of the batters have been used.

Eggplant Caponata

What you need:

- Red wine vinegar, 2 tbsp
- Bay leaf
- Capers, 3 tbsp
- White sugar, 2 tbsp
- Dry red wine, .33 c
- Water, 1 c
- Minced garlic, 3 cloves
- Fire-roasted tomatoes, 14.5 oz
- Dried oregano, 1 tsp
- Pepper, .5 tsp
- Cinnamon, .25 tsp
- Salt, .5 tsp
- Chopped onion
- Allspice, .25 tsp
- Diced small eggplant, 1 lb
- Olive oil, 2 tbsp

What you will do:

1. Add the oil into a skillet and let it heat up. Add in the spices, herbs, garlic, onion, and eggplant. Stir often, or until the onion has browned slightly. This will take around seven to eight minutes.

2. Turn the heat down a bit and mix in the bay leaf, wine, water, and tomatoes. Let this simmer, stirring often, until everything has become tender and it has started to thicken up. This will take about 13 to 15 minutes. Set it off of the heat and mix in the vinegar, capers, and sugar. Let it sit for 30 minutes and then take out the bay leaf. This should be served chilled or at room temp.

Tuna Artichoke Salad

What you need:

- Chopped red bell pepper
- Pepper, .5 tsp
- Tuna, 5 oz can
- Chopped spinach, 1 c
- Minced garlic, 2 cloves
- Olive oil, 1 tbsp
- Chopped dill, .25 c
- Lemon juice, 1 tbsp
- Chopped artichoke hearts, 6 oz jar

What you will do:

1. Stir together the pepper, garlic, lemon juice, oil, dill, and artichoke. Toss in the bell pepper, tuna, and spinach and toss it all together.

Black Beans and Quinoa

What you need:

- Chopped cilantro, .5 c
- Vegetable broth, 1.5 c
- Drained and rinsed black beans, 2 15-oz cans
- Frozen corn, 1 c
- Ground cumin, 1 tsp
- Pepper
- Cayenne pepper, .25 tsp
- Salt
- Quinoa, .75 c
- Chopped garlic, 3 cloves
- Chopped onion
- Vegetable oil, 1 tsp

What you will do:

1. Add the oil to a pot and add in the garlic and onion, cook until lightly browned.

2. Stir in the quinoa and then pour in the broth. Add the pepper, salt, cayenne, and cumin and then let everything come to a boil. Place the lid on the pot, turn the heat down, and let everything simmer until the quinoa is tender

and it has absorbed the broth. This takes about 20 minutes.

3. Mix the corn into and cook for five minutes more. Stir in the cilantro and black beans and enjoy.

Maples Salmon

What you need:

- Salmon, 1 lb
- Pepper
- Minced garlic, 1 clove
- Salt, .25 tsp
- Soy sauce, 2 tbsp
- Maple syrup

What you will do:

1. Stir together the pepper, salt, garlic, soy sauce, and maple syrup. Lay the salmon into a baking dish and cover with the syrup mixture. Place the lid on the dish and let it refrigerate for 30 minutes. Flip it halfway through.

2. Set your oven to 400. Cook the salmon for 20 minutes, uncovered, or until it can easily be flaked apart with a fork.

Balsamic Chicken

What you need:

- Dried Thyme, .5 tsp
- Dried rosemary, 1 tsp
- Dried oregano, 1 tsp
- Dried basil, 1 tsp
- Garlic salt, 1 tsp
- Balsamic vinegar, .5 c
- Pepper
- Can diced tomatoes, 14.5 oz
- Thinly sliced onion
- Olive oil, 2 tbsp
- Boneless, skinless chicken breast halves, 6

What you will do:

1. Rub the chicken with the pepper and garlic salt. Add the oil to a pan. Add in the chicken and brown each side, about three to four minutes on each side. Add in the onion. Cook and stir everything together until the onion has turned brown about three to four minutes.

2. Add in the balsamic vinegar and diced tomatoes. Add in the thyme, rosemary, oregano, and basil. Let everything simmer for about 15 minutes, or until the chicken is no longer pink. Enjoy.

Honey Mustard Chicken

What you need:

- Dried parsley, .5 tsp
- Paprika, 1 tsp
- Dried basil, 1 tsp
- Mustard, .5 c
- Honey, .5 c
- Pepper
- Salt
- Boneless, skinless chicken breast halves, 6

What you will do:

1. Start by heating your oven to 350.

2. Rub the chicken with the pepper and salt and then place them in a greased casserole dish. Mix the remaining ingredients together. Cover the chicken with half of the mixture.

3. Let it bake for 30 minutes. Flip the chicken and coat the other side with the rest of the mixture. Bake for 10 to 15 minutes more. It should reach 165. Let it rest for ten minutes.

Ginger Mahi Mahi

What you need:

- Olive oil, 2 tsp
- Crushed garlic, 1 clove
- Grated ginger, 1 tsp
- Balsamic vinegar, 3 tbsp
- Soy sauce, 3 tbsp
- Honey, 3 tbsp
- Vegetable oil, 1 tbsp
- Pepper
- Salt
- Mahi Mahi, 4 6-oz fillets

What you will do:

1. Mix the olive oil, garlic, ginger, balsamic vinegar, soy sauce, and honey together. Rub the fish with the pepper and salt and lay them in a baking dish. Pour the honey mixture over the top. Make sure the fish is skin-side down if it has a skin. Let this refrigerate for 20 minutes.

2. Add the vegetable oil to a pan. Reserve the marinade. Place the fish in the pan and fry four to six minutes on both sides. Turn the fish only once. Place on a platter and keep them warm.

3. Add the marinade into the pan and cook until the marinade has reduced to the consistency of a glaze. Spoon the glaze over top of the fish and enjoy it.

Chicken and Asparagus Penne

What you need:

- Low-sodium chicken broth, .5 c
- Garlic powder
- Pepper
- Salt
- Cubed chicken breasts, 2 halves
- Olive oil, 5 tbsp – divided
- Penne pasta, 16 oz
- Parmesan cheese, .25 c
- Thinly sliced garlic, 1 clove
- Sliced asparagus, 1 bunch

What you will do:

1. Fill a pot with water and add some salt. Let it boil. Add in the pasta and cook until it becomes al dente. This takes about eight to ten minutes. Drain out the water and set the pasta to the side

2. Add three tablespoons of the oil into a pan and add in the chicken. Sprinkle in some garlic powder, pepper, and salt. Mix everything together so the chicken is coated well. Cook the chicken until browned. This will take about five minutes. Set the chicken out on paper towels to drain.

3. Add the broth to the skillet and add in the garlic, asparagus, and a bit more pepper, garlic powder, and salt. Cover with a lid and let the asparagus steam until it has become tender. This will take about five to ten minutes. Add the chicken back in to warm through.

4. Add the chicken mixture into the pasta and stir everything together. Let it all sit together for about five minutes. Add in the remaining oil and the parmesan. Stir everything together and enjoy it.

Pest Chicken Florentine

What you need:

- Pesto, 2 tbsp
- Dry Alfredo mix, 4.5 oz package
- Spinach leaves, 2 c
- Sliced boneless skinless chicken breast halves, 4
- Chopped garlic, 1 clove
- Olive oil, 2 tbsp
- Grated Romano cheese, 1 tbsp
- Dry penne pasta, 8 oz package

What you will do:

1. Add the oil to a skillet and once heated, add in the garlic. Stir constantly for about a minute so the garlic doesn't burn. Stir in the chicken and cook for seven to eight minutes. Once the chicken is almost cooked, mix in the spinach and cook for three to four minutes more.

2. As that cook, fix the Alfredo sauce following the directions on the package. Once mixed, stir in the pesto.

3. Add the penne to a large pot of boiling water. Cook it for eight to ten minutes. Drain and rinse the pasta in cold water until cooled off.

4. Pour the spinach and chicken mixture into the pasta and then pour in the sauce mixture. Stir everything well and top with the cheese.

Chicken Tortilla Soup

What you need:

- Drained can diced tomatoes with green chile peppers, 10 oz
- Black beans, 15 oz can
- Chunk chicken, 10 oz can
- Chicken broth, 2 14.5-oz can
- Whole kernel corn, 15 oz can

What you will do:

1. Add all of the cans into a pot. Let them simmer together until everything is heated through. You can taste and add any other seasonings that you would like.

Turkey Chili

What you need:

- Minced garlic, 1 tbsp
- Mashed kidney beans, 16 oz
- Canned crushed tomatoes, 28 oz
- Water, 2 c
- Chopped onion
- Ground turkey, 1 lb
- Olive oil, 1.5 tsp
- Pepper, .5 tsp
- Salt, .5 tsp
- Cumin, .5 tsp
- Cayenne pepper, .5
- Dried oregano, .5 tsp
- Paprika, .5 tsp
- Chili powder, 2 tbsp

What you will do:

1. Add the oil to a pot and add in the turkey to the pot. Cook the turkey, breaking it apart until it has browned up. Mix in the onion, cooking until the onion is tender.

2. Add the water in and stir in the garlic, kidney beans, and tomatoes. Add in the herbs and spices. Let everything come up to a boil. Turn the heat down, place on the lid, and let it simmer for 30 minutes.

Amazing Chicken

What you need:

- Olive oil, 6 tbsp
- Pepper
- Salt, 1.5 tsp
- Brown sugar, .5 c
- Juice lemon, .5
- Juiced lime
- Minced garlic, 3 cloves
- Mustard, 3 tbsp
- Apple cider vinegar, .25 c
- Boneless, skinless chicken breast halves, 6

What you will do:

1. Mix together the pepper, brown sugar, lemon juice, salt, lime juice, garlic, mustard, and vinegar. Slowly mix in the oil. Place the chicken in the marinade and let it sit for eight hours in the fridge.

2. If you have a grill, heat the grill to high. You can also pan-fry these in a cast-iron skillet. Cook the chicken six to eight minutes on both sides, or until it comes up to the correct temperature. Discard the rest of the marinade.

Chicken with Orzo

What you need:

- Grated parmesan
- Spinach, 2 c
- Chopped parsley, 1 tbsp
- Salt
- Diced chicken breast halves, 2
- Crushed red pepper, .25 tsp
- Garlic, 2 cloves
- Olive oil, 2 tbsp
- Uncooked orzo, 1 c

What you will do:

1. Add water to a pot and let it come up to a boil. Add in the orzo and let it cook for eight to ten minutes. Drain and set to the side.

2. Add the oil to a pan and add in the red pepper and garlic, cooking for a few minutes. Mix in the chicken and sprinkle in some salt. Cook this for two to five minutes, or until the chicken is browned and the juices come out clear. Turn the heat down and stir in the orzo and parsley. Toss in the skillet. Stir occasionally, cooking for another five minutes or until the spinach has wilted. Serve topped with the parmesan.

Chicken Burrito

What you need:

- Hot sauce
- Chili powder, 1 tsp
- Minced garlic, 2 cloves
- Cumin, 1 tsp
- Taco seasoning packet
- Salsa, .25 c
- Tomato sauce, 4 oz
- Boneless, skinless chicken breast halves, 2
- Tortillas, 4

What you will do:

1. Add the tomato sauce and chicken to a pot. Let it come up to boil and then mix in the salsa, chili powder, garlic, and seasoning packet. Allow this all to simmer for 15 minutes.

2. Use a fork to pull the chicken apart. Continue to cook, lidded, for five to ten minutes. Mix in the hot sauce, adding enough for your taste. If the mixture is too thick, you can add a bit of water. Serve the filling on a tortilla.

Garlic Shrimp Linguine

What you need:

- Parsley, 1 tsp
- Pepper
- Salt
- Minced garlic, 3 cloves
- Grated parmesan, 2 tsp
- White wine, 3 tbsp
- Butter, 1 tbsp
- Linguine, 1 lb
- Cleaned medium shrimp, 1 lb

What you will do:

1. Add water to a pot and let it come to a boil. Add in the pasta and cook it for eight to ten minutes. Drain the water off.

2. In another pot, add the butter and once melted, mix in the pepper, parsley, salt, garlic, cheese, and wine. Let this simmer for three to five minutes, stirring often. Turn the heat up and then add in the shrimp. Let this cook for three to four minutes or until the shrimp have cooked through.

3. Divide out the pasta and top with the sauce. Sprinkle on some parmesan and parsley if desired.

Chickpea Salad

What you need:

- Pepper
- Salt
- Dried dill, 1 tsp
- Lemon juice, 1 tbsp
- Mayonnaise, 1 tbsp
- Chopped onion, .5
- Chopped celery, 1 stalk
- Rinsed garbanzo beans, 19 oz

What you will do:

1. Add the chickpeas to a bowl and mash them up a bit with a fork. Stir in the rest of the ingredients, adjusting the pepper and salt for your taste.

Greek Chicken Pasta Salad

What you need:

- Dried oregano, 2 tsp
- Pepper
- Lemon juice, 2 tbsp
- Salt
- Chopped parsley, 3 tbsp
- Crumbled feta, .5 c
- Chopped tomato
- Drained and chopped marinated artichoke hearts, 14 oz
- Diced chicken breast, 1 lb
- Crushed garlic, 2 cloves
- Olive oil, 1 tbsp
- Chopped red onion, .5 c
- Linguine pasta, 16 oz

What you will do:

1. Add water to a pot and let it come to a boil. Add in the pasta and cook for eight to ten minutes. Drain off the water.

2. Add the oil to a pan. Add in the garlic and onion, cooking for about two minutes. Mix in the chicken, stirring occasionally, until the chicken is cooked through. This will take about five to six minutes depending on how small you cut the chicken.

3. Turn the heat down, and mix in the pasta, oregano, lemon juice, parsley, feta, tomato, and artichoke hearts. Cook for two to three minutes. Set off the heat and mix in some pepper and salt. Serve with some lemon wedges.

Spicy Chicken

What you need:

- Boneless, skinless chicken breast halves, 4
- Pepper, 1 tbsp
- Cayenne pepper, 1 tbsp
- Dried thyme, 1 tbsp
- Onion powder, 1 tbsp
- Salt, 1 tbsp
- Garlic powder, 2 tbsp
- Paprika, 2.5 tbsp

What you will do:

1. Stir together all of the spices. Remove three tablespoons of the mixture. Keep the rest stored to use later on.

2. Rub the chicken with the reserved spice mixture. Heat up your grill or a skillet. Lightly oil them and then cook the chicken for about six to eight minutes on both sides, or until the chicken is cooked through. Enjoy.

Fra Diavolo

What you need:

- Chopped parsley, 1 tbsp
- Scallops, 8 oz
- Cleaned small shrimp, 8 oz
- Linguine, 16 oz
- Red pepper flakes, 1 tsp
- Salt, 1.5 tsp
- Chopped whole peeled tomatoes with their liquid, 3 c
- Crushed garlic, 6 cloves
- Olive oil, 4 tbsp - divided

What you will do:

1. Add two tablespoons of the oil to a pot and add in the garlic. Once the garlic begins sizzling, add in the tomatoes. Sprinkle in the red pepper flakes and the salt. Let this come up to a boil. Turn the heat down and let it simmer for 30 minutes.

2. As that cooks, fill another pot with water and let it come up to a boil. Add the pasta in and let it cook for eight to ten minutes. Drain the water off.

3. Add the rest of the oil to a skillet and then add in the scallops and shrimp. Let this cook for two minutes, stirring often. Once the shrimp turns pink, add them and the scallops to the tomato sauce. Mix in the parsley and cook for another three to four minutes. Serve this over the cooked pasta.

Pineapple Chicken

What you need:

- Skewers
- Chicken breast tenderloins, 2 lbs
- Low-sodium soy sauce, .33 c
- Brown sugar, .5 c
- Pineapple juice, 1 c

What you will do:

1. Add the soy sauce, brown sugar, and juice to a pot. Let it heat and then set it off the heat right before it starts to boil.

2. Add the chicken to a bowl and pour in the marinade you just made. Let this refrigerate for 30 minutes or more. Let the skewers, if wooden, soak in water while the chicken marinates.

3. Thread the chicken onto the skewers. Heat your grill up and lightly oil the grates. Place the skewers on the grill and cook for five minutes on both sides, or until it is cooked through.

Baked Halibut

What you need:

- Diced tomatoes, 2 c
- Minced garlic, 1 clove
- Minced onion, .5 c
- Diced zucchini, 1 c
- Olive oil, 1 tsp
- Crumbled feta, .33 c
- Halibut steaks, 4 6-oz steaks
- Pepper, .25 tsp
- Salt, .25 tsp
- Chopped basil, 2 tbsp

What you will do:

1. Start by setting your oven to 450. Grease a casserole dish and set it to the side.

2. Add the oil to a pot and add in the garlic, onion, and zucchini. Let this cook for about five minutes, or until everything is tender. Set off the heat and then stir in the pepper, salt, basil, and tomatoes.

3. Place the halibut in the casserole dish. Divide the veggie mixture over top of the steaks. Sprinkle on the feat.

4. Place this in the oven and cook for 15 minutes, or until the fish easily flakes apart.

Not Tuna Salad

What you need:

- Pepper
- Salt
- Chopped green onions, 2
- Sweet pickle relish, 1 tbsp
- Spicy brown mustard, 2 tsp
- Mayonnaise, 2 tbsp
- Mashed garbanzo beans, 19 oz

What you will do:

1. Place all of the ingredients into a bowl and mix them together. Serve as is or on bread as a sandwich.

Turkey Meatloaf Cups

What you need:

- Egg
- Uncooked Couscous, .5 c
- Extra lean ground turkey, 1 lb
- Chopped red bell pepper
- Chopped onion, 1.5 c
- Chopped zucchini, 2 c
- Barbecues sauce, .5 c
- Dijon mustard, 1 tbsp
- Worcestershire sauce, 2 tbsp

What you will do:

1. Start by setting your oven to 400. Grease 20 muffin tin cups with nonstick spray.

2. Place the bell pepper, onion, and zucchini in a food processor and pulse until they are finely chopped. Place in a bowl along with the mustard, Worcestershire sauce, egg, couscous, and turkey. Mix everything together until well combined. Add the mixture to the muffin cup, filling ¾ of the way full. Place a teaspoon of the barbecues sauce to the top of each.

3. Bake for about 25 minutes. The muffin cups should reach 160. Allow them to sit for about five minutes before removing and serving.

Kale and Bean Soup

What you need:

- Chopped plum tomatoes, 4
- Undrained white beans, 2 15-oz cans
- Low-sodium vegetable broth, 4 c
- Chopped kale, 4 c
- Chopped onion
- Minced garlic, 8 cloves
- Olive oil, 1 tbsp
- Chopped parsley, 1 c
- Pepper
- Salt
- Italian herb seasoning, 2 tsp

What you will do:

1. Place the oil in a pot and add in the onion and garlic. Cook until they become soft. Add in the kale, stirring until it has wilted. Mix in the pepper, salt, herbs, tomatoes, 2 cups of beans, and 3 cups of broth. Let this all simmer together for about five minutes. Using a blender, add in the remaining beans and broth, mixing until smooth. Add this into the soup and stir together. This will help thicken it. Cook everything together for another 15 minutes. Enjoy with a sprinkling of chopped parsley.

Black Bean Chili

What you need:

- Chili powder, 1.5 tbsp
- Crushed tomatoes, 14.5 oz
- Undrained black beans, 3 15-oz cans
- Ground turkey, 1 lb
- Minced garlic, 2 cloves
- Diced onion
- Vegetable oil, 1 tbsp
- Red wine vinegar, 1 tbsp
- Dried basil leaves, 1 tbsp
- Dried oregano, 1 tbsp

What you will do:

1. Add the oil to a pot and then add in the garlic and onion, cooking until the onion becomes translucent. Add in the turkey, and cook until it is browned. Mix in the vinegar, basil, oregano, chili powder, tomatoes, and beans. Lower the heat, and then let it simmer for 60 minutes. Stir and again and enjoy it.

Teriyaki Chicken

What you need:

- Sesame oil, 2 tsp
- Minced garlic, 2 tsp
- Lemon juice, .25 c
- Teriyaki sauce, 1 c
- Boneless, skinless chicken breast halves, 4

What you will do:

1. Add the oil, garlic, lemon juice, teriyaki sauce, and chicken in a bag. Close the bag and shake everything together so that the chicken is well coated. Let this refrigerate for 24 hours, shaking the bag every couple of hours.

2. Heat up your grill to high.

3. Grease the grill with some oil and place the chicken on the heated grill. Discard the rest of the marinade. Cook the chicken on both sides for six to eight minutes. The juices should be clear and the temp should get to 165.

Peanut Chicken

What you need:

- Boneless, skinless chicken breast halves, 4
- Cayenne pepper, dash
- Curry powder, .33 tsp
- Chopped garlic clove
- Soy sauce, 2 tsp
- Lime juice, 1 tbsp
- Peanut butter, 2 tbsp

What you will do:

1. Heat up your grill to high.
2. Mix the pepper, curry, garlic, soy sauce, lime juice, and peanut butter together. Oil the grill and lay the chicken on. Brush the top sides of the chicken with half of the sauce. Allow them to cook for six to eight minutes. Flip the chicken over and brush the other side with the rest of the sauce. Grill for another six to eight minutes. Enjoy.

Tuna Patties

What you need:

- Vegetable oil, 2 tbsp
- Cornmeal, .5 c
- Pepper, 1 tsp
- Sesame oil, 1 tsp
- Ketchup, 1 tbsp
- Teriyaki sauce, 1 tbsp
- Soy sauce, 1 tbsp
- Minced garlic, 1 clove
- Minced green onions, 3
- Bread crumbs, .75 c
- Beaten egg
- Tuna, 2 5-oz cans

What you will do:

1. Mix the garlic, onion, bread crumbs, egg, and tuna together in a bowl. Whisk the pepper, oil, ketchup, teriyaki, and soy sauce together. Pour this into the tuna mixture and stir together. Form the tuna in six patties. Sprinkle the sides with some cornmeal.

2. Add the oil to a pan and then lightly fry each patty about five minutes on both sides.

Jerk Chicken

What you need:

- Sliced boneless, skinless chicken breast halves, 4

- Sliced habanero pepper

- Allspice, .5 tsp

- Chopped garlic, 3 cloves

- Sesame oil, 1 tsp

- Chopped thyme, 2 tsp

- Red wine vinegar, 4 tbsp

- Soy sauce, 4 tbsp

- Brown sugar, 3 tbsp

- Finely chopped onion, 1 tsp

What you will do:

1. Add the pepper, allspice, garlic, sesame oil, thyme, vinegar, soy sauce, brown sugar, and onion to a blender and mix until smooth. Add the chicken to a bag and pour in ¾ of the sauce. Shake everything around and let it marinate for at least an hour.

2. Heat up the broiler in your oven.

3. Take the chicken out, getting rid of the extra marinade. Place the chicken on a broiler pan and cook for 10 to 15 minutes, flipping once. Add the reaming sauce to a pot and heat. Pour this over the chicken for serving.

Broccoli Soup

What you need:

- Chicken broth, 4 c
- Chopped and peeled potato
- Chopped frozen broccoli, 2 10-oz packages
- Chopped garlic, 3 cloves
- Chopped onion
- Olive oil, 1 tbsp
- Pepper
- Nutmeg, .25 tsp
- Salt

What you will do:

1. Add the oil to a pot and then add in the garlic and onion, cooking until soft. Mix in the chicken broth, potato, and broccoli. Let this come up to a boil and then turn the heat down to a simmer. Let it cook for 15 minutes, or until everything is tender.

2. Using an immersion blender, puree everything until smooth. Place it back over the heat and heat everything through. Add some pepper, nutmeg, and salt to taste.

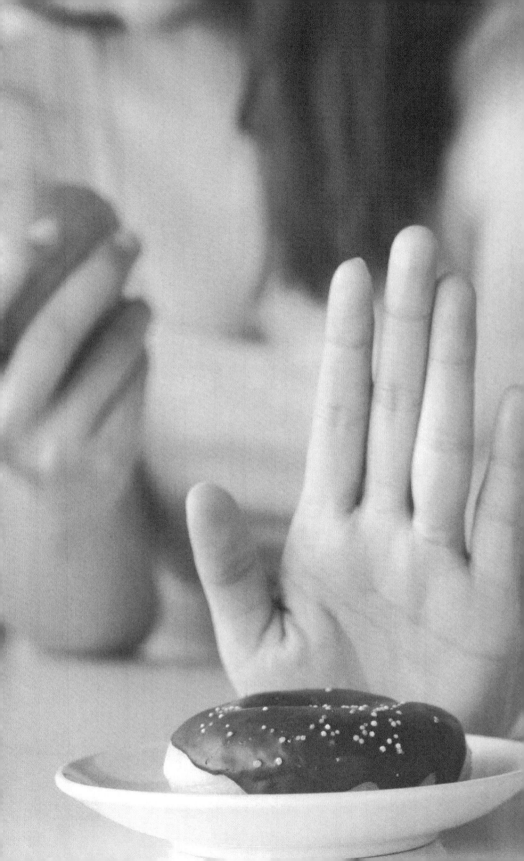

WEEKLY PLAN

One of the best ways to make sure that you stick to a new diet or eating schedule is to create a weekly plan. When you know what meals you are having and when, it's pretty hard to talk yourself into grabbing McDonald's on the way home.

We'll start by looking at how to create your own weekly meal plan, and then I will provide you with a meal plan for one week to get you started.

Planning Your Meals

To start, you will want to figure out what meals you want to have during the coming week. Once you have figured that out, you can write down your grocery list. When you buy for the week, it will mean that you won't have to make as many shopping trips during the week. Here are some tips:

1. Take a look to see what you already have. Check your fridge, freezer, and cabinets. Write down or remember the things that you already have on hand. You will save money if you use these things in the coming week instead of buying all new things.

2. Create a worksheet to help you plan out your meals. You can get fancy and make a spreadsheet using Microsoft, or you can simply write something out on a piece of paper. Keeping it on your fridge for the week will serve as a reminder for what you are supposed to be doing.

3. Write down a list of recipes that you would like to try. Try to find some new, healthy ideas that you can make with food you have on hand, and would be fun for the entire family to try.

4. Take a look at your schedule and see what you will be able to cook. Pick meals that can easily be prepared on days where you will be busy. Then you can choose things that are more time consuming on days where you don't have a lot going on. Slow cooker meals are a great idea for busy days as well.

5. Make a plan to use up your leftovers as well. You don't have to cook every single day. Using leftovers will save you time and money.

Now, you should be able to come up with your own weekly meal plans with ease. Don't forget to schedule your fasting times as well.

One Week Meal Plan

With this one-week meal plan, we will be easing you into a 16/8 schedule. It will start with your feeding and fasting times both being at 12 and then your fasting window will grow each day until you reach 16/8.

- Day One: Fast for 12 hours, Eat for 12 hours.

o Meal One – Chia Pudding

o Meal Two – Chicken Salad

o Meal Three – Chicken Chili

o You can have a snack between meals if you feel that you need one.

- Day Two: Fast for 13 hours, Eat for 11 hours

o Meal One – Protein Shake

o Meal Two – Chickpea Salad

o Meal Three – Quinoa Salad

o Again, you can have a snack if you need to

- Day Three: Fast for 14 hours, Eat for 10

o Meal One – Protein Shake

o Meal Two – Leftovers from meal three on day one

o Meal Three – Tuna Salad Sandwiches

o After today, you will be down to two meals and a snack

- Day Four: Fast for 15 hours, Eat for 9

o Meal One – Egg Muffin

o Snack – Piece of Fruit

o Meal Two – Leftovers from meal three on day two

- Day Five: Fast for 16 hours, Eat for 8

o Meal One – Veggie Omelet

o Snack – Boiled egg

o Meal Two – Chicken Salad

- Day Six: Fast for 16 hours, Eat for 8

o Meal One – Leftover chicken salad from the day before

o Snack – Trail mix

o Meal Two – Leftover quinoa salad

- Day Seven: Fast for 16 hours, Eat for 8

o Meal One – Protein Smoothie

o Snack – Carrots and hummus

o Meal Two – Avocado chickpea salad

This is just a simple meal plan. You can make yours however you would like, and if you would prefer to have three tiny meals during your eating time, then feel free. The most important thing is to eat smart and abide by your eating and fasting windows.

IF FOR WOMEN

Women are often the ones who have a hard time figuring out a safe way to intermittent fast. Some women will experience missed periods, metabolic problems, and, in rare cases, early-onset menopause. Women can intermittent fast safely, but it is important to look at what can happen if it isn't followed properly.

The hormones that control functions like ovulation are sensitive to energy intake. The hypothalamic-pituitary-gonadal axis works similarly to an air traffic controller. The hypothalamus starts things off by releasing the gonadotropin-releasing hormone. This shoots a message over to the pituitary gland to release follicular stimulating hormone and luteinizing hormone. Both of these hormones act on the gonads, which are the ovaries or testes. For a woman, this will trigger the production of progesterone and estrogen. In men, it will trigger the production of sperm and testosterone.

For some women, a short fast can end up altering these hormones. Some people believe that missing a single meal can cause a woman's body to go on high alert. This gives the body the change to respond quickly to change in energy consumption. This might be why some women aren't affected by fasting but others are.

Nobody is really sure as to why women's hormones tend to be more affected than men's. But one possibility is kisspeptin. This is a protein-like molecule that assists neurons in talking with each other. Kisspeptin stimulates GnRH and is extremely sensitive to ghrelin, insulin, and leptin, which also react to and regulate satiety and hunger.

Females, in all mammal species, tend to have more kisspeptin. With more kisspeptin, it can create more sensitivity to changes in energy levels. This might be one reason why fasting causes the kisspeptin levels in women to drop and then causes GnRH to be knocked off-kilter.

You may be thinking, what is so bad about skipping some periods? I'm not planning to have kids anytime soon.

Things aren't that simple. The reproductive system and metabolism are very closely intertwined. If you were to start skipping periods, you probably have some messed up hormones and not just the ones that affect getting pregnant.

Women often eat less protein than men. When fasting, women are going to consume even less. When you eat less protein, then your body has fewer amino acids.

Amino acids activate the estrogen receptors and synthesize IGF-1 within the liver. IGF-1 triggers the thickening of the uterine lining and helps it to move through the reproductive cycle. This is why low-protein diets can hurt a woman's fertility.

Estrogen doesn't just help with reproduction either. Your body had lots of estrogen receptors, including in the brain, GI tract, and bones. If you mess up your estrogen balance, the metabolic functions will change, which includes bone formation, protein turnover, cognition, recovery, moods, digestion, and so on.

Estrogen does many different things when it comes to energy and appetite. First, estrogen will modify the peptides that send signals to the brain to tell you if you are hungry or full. Then the estrogen stimulates neurons in the hypothalamus that stop the production of appetite-regulating peptides.

If estrogen levels drop too low, it could make you feel hungrier. Estrogen plays a very important part as a metabolic regulator. This probably seems very unfair. Men just think about losing weight, and it happens. But women can do crunches all day long and nothing happens. But, if you look at it from an evolutionary standpoint, women don't really need to have washboard abs.

The human female is a very unique mammal. Every other mammal has the ability to pause or terminate pregnancies whenever they want. Female humans can't do this. For female humans, the placenta takes over and the fetus takes control of the body.

The baby controls the insulin in the mother so that it can take more glucose. The fetus can also dilate the blood vessels in the mother, and change your blood pressure so that it can get more nutrients.

The baby has one thought, and that is to survive no matter what it does to the mother. This is what is called a "maternal-fetal conflict," and many scientists compare this to the host-virus relationship. A woman can't simply ask the fetus to stop growing because food is in low amounts. So, if a woman were to be fertile during a famine, it could prove to be very fatal. This is the reason why the reproduction pathways in women are extremely sensitive to metabolic changes.

This means that there is a chance that intermittent fasting can affect the reproductive health of a woman if the body thinks it is a threat. Anything that has the ability to affect your reproductive health has the possibility of affecting your overall health and fitness. But as you already know, intermittent fasting comes in many different shapes and sizes.

Women, you don't have to give up on intermittent fasting. It does mean, though, that you need to take things a little more cautiously. First off, if you start to feel any of these systems, you need to stop your fasting:

- You are constantly cold.

- You start having trouble digesting things.

- You have a low sexual desire, and when you do have sex, your lady parts aren't into it.

- You notice that your heart is beating differently.

- You start having extreme mood swings.

- You don't handle stress as well as you used to.

- You get sick a lot or you heal from injuries slowly.

- Your body takes longer to recover from workouts.

- You start developing acne or your skin becomes really dry.

- You start losing your hair.

- You have a hard time getting to sleep or staying asleep.

- Your menstrual cycle becomes irregular or quits altogether.

As far as pregnant women go, you should avoid experimenting with fasting because your body has higher energy requirements. If you tend to be under a great deal of stress, fasting might not be good on your body.

Fasting Safely

As we know, fasting can cause a lot of problems for women, especially if they are new to it or jump into fasting too quickly. For women that want to start intermittent fasting, using crescendo intermittent fasting might be a good idea.

With this schedule of fasting, you will only fast a few days of the week instead of every single day. This will prevent women from throwing themselves into a hormonal frenzy while also benefiting from fasting. This is a gentler approach that will help your body to adapt to fasting. When you do this correctly, it is one of the best ways to lose weight, gain more energy, and improve inflammatory markers.

Not every single woman will find it necessary to try crescendo fasting, but this can help to ensure success for most women. Here's how you do it:

1. The fasting windows will first happen on two to three nonconsecutive days, like Monday, Wednesday, and Friday.

2. When you do fast, do light cardio or yoga.

3. Ideally, the fasting times on those days should be 12 to 16 hours long.

4. On the other days of the weeks, you can eat normally and perform intense workouts and strength training.

5. Make sure that you drink plenty of water. Coffee and tea are perfectly fine, as long as you leave out the milk and sweetener.

6. Once you have followed this schedule for two weeks, you can then add another day of fasting. This means you will have two days of fasting back to back.

On the fasting days, you will still eat, it will just follow the 16/8 schedule. Using the crescendo method, you slowly ease your way into a 16/8 protocol. It is not a good idea for women to try the 5:2 schedule or any of the others that would mean that you have to fast for 24 hours. If you were to try an eat-stop-eat schedule, you should only do the fasting days twice a week.

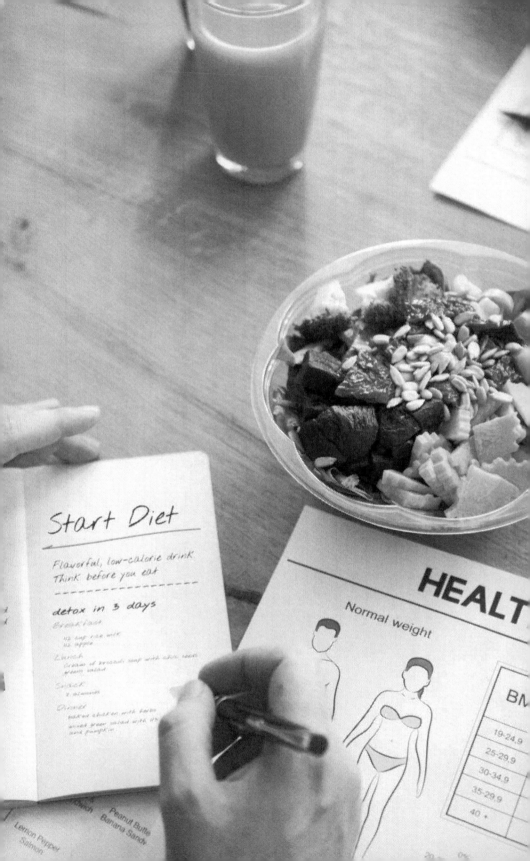

IF WITH FITNESS

One thing that most people worry about when fasting is if they can exercise. They worry that they won't have the energy. Won't intermittent fasting hurt your energy levels? The most important thing to remember is that timing is the most important thing. When you do and don't eat will impact the type of workout you do.

There is a research that has found that when in a fasted stated, fat oxidation and lipolysis increase. The stomach will receive extra blood flow, and this is the hardest region to lose weight. Fasting aids in weight loss in this area.

No matter what workout you are doing, the body will use stored carbs or glycogen as fuel. The main exception is when your glycogen reserves become depleted. This might happen if you have been fasting for a while. If this happens, then your body will have to find different things to burn for energy, such as fat. One study has found that men who ran before breakfast would burn 20% more fat than people who made sure they ate before.

It's not fun trying to push through a workout when you are hungry, though. So the important thing is to sweat smart when you are fasting.

Sweating Smart

When you are fasting, and you want to exercise, which you should, the following are some ways to make sure that you get the most from your exercise without causing harm.

- When you exercise.

There are three different times that you can choose from when you are fasting. You will need to figure out if you should exercise before, after, or during your eating time.

Working out before you have your first meal is good for people who do well exercising with an empty stomach. Exercising in the middle of your eating time is good if you tend to get woozy when exercising on an empty stomach. To get the best performance and recovery, exercising in the middle of your eating window is the way to go.

Exercising at the end of your eating window is a good idea for people who want to have fuel for their workout, but is okay with not having a post-workout meal. Keep in mind, there is a chance that you might start feeling hungry before you are supposed to eat.

- Think about your macronutrients to figure out your workout.

While counting your macronutrients isn't necessary unless you are following a keto diet, you can still keep track of them on the days before your workout days. On the days you plan on strength training, you will want to consume more carbs that day. You can do cardio and HIIT training on days you eat fewer carbs.

If you are able to, try to do intense or moderate workouts shortly after your last meal of the day. When you do this, you will have plenty of glycogen to help fuel you. It also keeps you from ending up with low blood sugar. When you do high-intensity workouts, you will want to have a light snack after to help your muscles recover.

- Try to figure out your intensity level.

To figure out how intense you are working out, pay attention to how hard you are breathing. You want to make sure that if you are exercising in a fasted state that you can still carry a conversation.

- Have a high-protein meal.

If you are looking to build or keep your muscle mass, you will want to eat protein-heavy meals before and after weight training. Consuming protein on a regular basis is important for muscle synthesis.

- Healthy snacks are important.

Remember, during your eating time, you can eat whatever you want. Take advantage of this by having a snack a couple of hours before your workout, or shortly after your workout. Peanut butter toast with a banana is a good choice.

- Make sure you stay hydrated.

When you are fasting, you should still be drinking plenty of water. You should actually be drinking more water during your fasting window. And if you are working out while fasting, make sure you keep water close by.

- Listen to what your body is telling you.

The best piece of exercise advice that I can give you is to listen to your body. Your body knows what it can and can't do, so listen to it. If you start feeling weak or dizzy, stop. You may be experiencing low blood sugar or dehydration. If this happens, then you may need to make sure you eat before you workout.

People can and should work out when following an intermittent fasting schedule. Whether you choose to work out during your fasted or fed state is up to you and your body. Some people feel working out while fasted makes them feel better; others, not so much. Do what works best for you.

FAQ

While most of your questions should have already been answered throughout this book, to make sure, I have provided some common questions about intermittent fasting. This will ensure that you know exactly what you should do.

1. Who can safely intermittent fast?

Anybody can choose to intermittent fast as long as they are in reasonable health. If you are serious about taking control of your health, intermittent fasting can help. If your diabetes isn't currently being regulated, you need to speak with your doctor and get things under control before you start fasting. Women who are breastfeeding or pregnant might not want to fast. People who are underweight or have a history of eating disorders should avoid fasting.

2. What do I need to take into consideration before I begin a fasting schedule?

Take a look at your current routine, your work, your bodily limitations, and your habits when you are hungry or thirsty. The better you understand your life, the easier things will go. It also doesn't hurt to make sure that you understand the different schedules.

3. What do I need to think about if I have diabetes?

Make sure that you go into intermittent fasting cautiously. I wouldn't suggest trying some of the longer fasts. 16/8 is probably the safest option, and even still, you should ease yourself into it so that your body can adapt. Also, steer clear of heavy cardio workouts during fasting periods. There is a chance that fasting can create problems for diabetics, so make sure that you pay attention to your body, and if you need to, eat.

4. Can intermittent fasting help you with more than just losing weight?

Yes, it can. Fasting has the ability to help your mood, heart, brain, digestive system, and more. Many people choose to start fasting for these benefits rather than weight loss.

5. What is the best schedule to go with?

I can't answer this question for you. This is very subject, and it depends on the person. Everybody is going to have to decide which schedule works best for them.

6. Where is the best place to start with intermittent fasting?

Do more research. While this book has quite a bit of information, it still doesn't hurt to read more books and blogs about the subject. Getting more information never hurts anybody.

7. I am currently breastfeeding. Should I fast or wait until I stop?

In general, it is best to wait until after you are finished breastfeeding. While breastfeeding, your body is trying to provide important nutrients to the baby, so it is better not to risk messing up that process. It might end up hurting you and you may not be able to give your baby the nutrients it needs. But, that being said, there are some women who do and they don't have any problems. You need to do your own research on this topic and do what you think is right for you.

8. Should I exercise while I am fasting?

Starting out, exercises should be kept at a minimum and should be low-impact. If you have been regularly doing intense exercises, you may notice that you aren't able to do as much. Begin small and then start to increase the intensity to see what you are able to do. Women and diabetics, while in their fasted state, should stay away from intense exercises.

9. Do I have to follow a certain diet when fasti g?

If you want to, you can. Many people find that most diets don't work well with IF except for a ketogenic diet. If you start trying to restrict your protein or fat intake while fasting, you may find that you get hungry faster. I suggest just eating a healthy and well-balanced diet. You shouldn't do anything strict, just sensible.

10. I started getting headaches after I started fasting, why?

This isn't something everybody experiences, but some do. This is most often caused by dehydration, but not always. Up your water intake and see if that solves the problem. If it doesn't, then the headache is likely caused by withdrawals. The more you fast, the less frequent these headaches will become.

11. Can I drink anything while fasting?

Yes, and you should. As long as it doesn't contain calories, you can have all you want. Water is the most important thing to have.

12. Can expecting mothers fast?

It is not recommended. Some people say it is fine, but it is probably best if you didn't. Your body needs a lot of nutrients and plenty of calories when pregnant so that the fetus receives all of the nutrients possible.

CONCLUSION

Thank you for making it through to the end of Intermittent Fasting Diabetes. Let's hope it was informative and able to provide you with all of the tools you need to achieve your goals whatever they may be.

Diabetes is completely reversible, and intermittent fasting is a great way to do just that. No monthly fees, no special foods, just a different eating schedule. It really couldn't get any easier. And when you first start, you might find it hard to fast for more than a few hours, but that's okay. You work to grow your fasting periods. So experiment with some of the schedules and figure out which one works best for you.

Often life is not easy. Often to get something we have to face hard tests and face ourselves first.

What gives us energy every day, what allows us to always get up and smile at life even in the midst of a thousand difficulties, must be the deep love and respect for ourselves and the people we love.

Being healthy is not only important for ourselves but also for them.

A better life comes only if we really want it and if we are willing to change.

So my best wishes for a healthy lifestyle!

Jason R.

Printed in Great Britain
by Amazon